Core Clinical Cases
Problem Based Learning
Self Assessment
for
Medical Students
Book 2

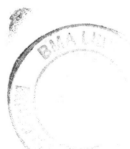

PasTest

Dedicated to y

Core Clinical Cases
Problem Based Learning
Self Assessment
for
Medical Students
Book 2

Andrew Sewart MB ChB

Foundation year 1 doctor

Royal Lancaster Infirmary

Lancaster

Henriette van Ruiten MB ChB

Foundation year 1 doctor

Royal Lancaster Infirmary

Lancaster

Edited by

Deborah Anne Wales MB ChB FRCP FRCA

Consultant Respiratory Physician

Nevill Hall Hospital

Abergavenny

Monmouthshire

© 2005 PASTEST LTD
Egerton Court
Parkgate Estate
Knutsford
Cheshire
WA16 8DX

Telephone: 01565 752000

First Published 2005
ISBN: 1904627560

PasTest Revision Books and Intensive Courses
PasTest has been established in the field of postgraduate medical education since
1972, providing revision books and intensive study courses for doctors preparing
for their professional examinations.

Books and courses are available for the following specialties:
MRCGP, MRCP Parts 1 and 2, MRCPCH Parts 1 and 2, MRCPsych, MRCS,
MRCOG Parts 1 and 2, DRCOG, DCH, FRCA, PLAB Parts 1 and 2.

For further details contact:
PasTest, Freepost, Knutsford, Cheshire WA16 7BR
Tel: 01565 752000 Fax: 01565 650264
www.pastest.co.uk enquiries@pastest.co.uk
Text prepared by Carnegie Publishing, Lancaster
Printed and bound in the UK by Athenaeum Press

DEDICATION

To all the FY1 doctors out there and those incessant bleeps, impossible veins, endless ward-rounds and not to mention the DOPs, mini-CEXs, CbDs, and mini-PATs (as if there were not enough acronyms already in medicine!).

CONTRIBUTORS

We would like to thank the following people for reviewing the cases within their specialty and for tactfully pointing out any glaring errors (of which there were a few!).

Dr. Jo Blair *MBChB, MRCP, MRCPCH, MD*
Consultant Paediatric Endocrinologist. Royal Liverpool Children's hospital.
Endocrine case 3

Mrs P. Brier *RN DipHE ENB 219, 998.*
Trainee Surgical Care Practitioner in Orthopaedics. Royal Lancaster Infirmary.
Surgical case 2

Mr T.A.J. Calvey *FRCS (Gen Surg)*
Consultant Surgeon. Royal Lancaster Infirmary.
Surgical cases 1, 3 and 4

Dr. Margaret Ellam *MBChB, FRCA*
Consultant in Palliative Medicine. Royal Lancaster Infirmary and St John's Hospice.
Palliative care case 1

Dr. D.W. Gorst *MA, BM BCh, FRCP, FRCPath*
Consultant Haematologist. Royal Lancaster Infirmary.
Haematology cases 1 and 2; palliative care case 2

Dr. P. Nardeosingh *MBBS, MRCP (UK), MRCPCH*
Associate Specialist in Paediatrics. Royal Lancaster Infirmary.
Paediatric cases 1 and 2

Dr. S Pidd *MBChB, FRSPsych*
Consultant in General Adult Psychiatry. Morecambe Bay Community Mental Health Team. Morecambe Bay Primary Care Trust.
Psychiatric cases 1 and 2

Mr B. Rhodes *MBBS, BSc, FRCS, FRCS (ortho)*
Consultant Orthopaedic Surgeon. Royal Lancaster Infirmary.
Surgical case 2

Mr R. Sinha *MBBS, MS (ortho), FRCS (Ed), FRCS (I)*
Trust Grade Surgeon in Orthopaedics. Royal Lancaster Infirmary.
Surgical case 2

Miss A. White *MBChB, MRCS*
Trust Grade Surgeon in Orthopaedics. Royal Lancaster Infirmary.
Surgical case 2

CONTENTS

FOREWORD

The authors of this book are newly qualified doctors in Year 1 of Foundation Training in the Morecambe Bay Trusts. Remarkably, this is their second book in the series. The first was completed whilst they were still undergraduates of the Medical School at the University of Liverpool. When they joined us in September 2003 at the start of their studies in year 4, they did so at a time when we were newcomers to the Liverpool curriculum. Little did they know how much they would teach their teachers and supervisors along the way.

This volume contains core cases in psychiatry, haematology, palliative care and emergency medicine which were not contained in the first book. The main difference though, and a matter of great pride to NHS staff in this area, is the list of contributors. Some are consultants, one is a colleague in Liverpool, others are non-consultant doctors and one is a nurse. This mix of contributors is a powerful affirmation of our commitment to interdisciplinary education and it arose quite spontaneously. The authors asked for help where they thought they might succeed and no-one refused. There was nothing contrived about this team.

It has been a matter of quiet pleasure to see the progress of the authors from students to colleagues. The steady application of effort in a worthy project has resulted in a valuable resource for students and teachers alike. We are proud and grateful to have them on our staff because they are instrumental in developing academic medical education in the new association between Liverpool University and the NHS in North Lancashire and Cumbria. I hope that you too will benefit from the fruit of their labours.

Dr Michael Flanagan
Director of Medical and Dental Education
Morecambe Bay NHS Trust
and
Undergraduate Sub-Dean
University of Liverpool

INTRODUCTION

When writing the first book of *Problem Based Learning: Core Clinical Cases* we always envisaged a second book to follow soon after. The range of core clinical cases that medical students are expected to be able to diagnose and manage is, as we are sure readers of this book will attest to, fairly daunting. The first book covered over sixty of these cases. This second book not only goes a long way to completing the list of core clinical cases, but also addresses those specialties which were not covered fully (or at all) in the first book. So, in this volume, for example, core surgical cases such as bowel cancer, peripheral vascular disease and breast cancer have been included. We have also included trauma cases such as head injury and hip fractures. Cases from specialties such as emergency medicine, psychiatry, endocrinology, haematology and neurology are included as well as those from palliative care, which is gaining increasing prominence in the undergraduate curriculum.

The format is the same as the first book; a series of questions prompts the reader through the diagnosis and management of each specific case with the addition of X-rays, CT scans, ECGs and blood results for added realism. However, in this volume, we have given greater emphasis to the accompanying teaching notes, with the aim of writing not only a self-assessment book but also a core reference book for your clinical attachments.

We were delighted with the success of the first book and hope you find this second book as equally helpful during your medical studies.

Andy and Henriette
Lancaster, September 2005.

NORMAL VALUES

Haematology

Haemoglobin	men:	13–18 g/dL
	women:	11.5–16 g/dL
Mean cell volume MCV		76–96 fL
Platelets		150–400 x 109/L
White cells (total)		4–11 x 109/L
INR		0.9–1.2

Arterial blood gases (ABGs)

pH	7.35–7.45
Po_2	10–12 kPa
Pco_2	4.7–6 kPa
HCO_3.	22–28 mmol/L
Base excess	±2 mmol/L

Urea and electrolytes (U&Es)

Sodium	135–145 mmol/L
Potassium	3.5–5 mmol/L
Creatinine	70–120 mmol/L
Urea	2.5–6.7 mmol/L
Albumin	35–50 g/L
Calcium	2.12–2.65 mmol/L
Phosphate	0.8–1.45 mmol/L

Liver function tests (LFTs)

Bilirubin	3–17 µmol/L
Alanine aminotransferase (ALT)	3–35 iu/L
Aspartate transaminase (AST)	3–35 iu/L
Alkaline phosphatase (ALP)	30–150 iu/L
gamma glutamyl transferase (γGT)	11–51 iu/L

Other biochemical values

Amylase	0–180 units/dL
Glucose, fasting	4–6 mmol/L
C-reactive protein (CRP)	<10 mg/L
TSH	0.5–5.7 mu/L
T_4 (thyroxine)	70–140 nmol/L
T_3 (tri-iodothyroxine)	1.2–3.0 nmol/L

ABBREVIATIONS

5FU	5-fluorouracil
5HT	5-hydroxytryptamine or serotonin
AAP	atypical antipsychotic
ABG	arterial blood gas
ABSPI	ankle–brachial systolic pressure index
ACE	angiotensin-converting enzyme
ACh	acetylcholine
ACR	albumin:creatinine ratio
ACS	acute coronary syndrome
ACTH	adrenocorticotrophic hormone
ADH	antidiuretic hormone
AFP	α-fetoprotein
AIDS	acquired immune deficiency syndrome
ALL	acute lymphoblastic leukaemia
ALP	alkaline phosphatase
ALT	alanine transaminase
AP	anteroposterior
ARDS	acute respiratory distress syndrome
AVN	avascular necrosis
AXR	abdominal X-ray
BCS	breast-conserving surgery
bd	twice daily
BE	base excess
BLS	basic life support
BMA	British Medical Association
BP	blood pressure
BPV	benign positional vertigo
CBT	cognitive behavioural therapy
CCU	coronary care unit
CHD	coronary heart disease
CLL	chronic lymphocytic leukaemia
CMF	cyclophosphamide, methotrexate, 5FU
CMV	cytomegalovirus
CNS	central nervous system
COC	combined oral contraceptive
COMT	catechol-O-methyl transferase

COPD	chronic obstructive pulmonary disease
CPR	cardiopulmonary resuscitation
CVP	cyclophosphamide, vincristine and prednisolone
CR	complete remission
CSF	cerebrospinal fluid
CT	computed tomography
CTZ	chemoreceptor trigger zone
CVA	cerebrovascular accident
CVD	cardiovascular disease
CVS	cardiovascular system
CXR	chest X-ray
DEXA	dual-energy X-ray absorptiometry
DHS	dynamic hip screw
DKA	diabetic ketoacidosis
DVT	deep vein thrombosis
EBV	Epstein–Barr virus
ECG	electrocardiogram
ECT	electroconvulsive therapy
EEG	electroencephalogram
EPSs	extrapyramidal symptoms
ER	oestrogen receptor
ESR	erythrocyte sedimentation rate
FBC	full blood count
FNA	fine-needle aspiration
FSH	follicle-stimulating hormone
FY1	foundation year 1
G-CSF	granulocyte colony-stimulating factor
GCS	Glasgow Coma Score
GH	growth hormone
GI	gastrointestinal
GORD	gastro-oesophageal reflux disease
GTN	glyceryl trinitrate
GVHD	graft-versus-host disease
Hb	haemoglobin
HbA1c	glycated haemoglobin
HDL	high-density lipoprotein
HIV	human immunodeficiency virus
HLA	human leukocyte antigen
HONK	hyperosmolar, non-ketotic

HR	heart rate
HRT	hormone replacement therapy
HSV	herpes simplex virus
IBD	inflammatory bowel disease
ICP	intracranial pressure
ICS	intercostal space
IF	intrinsic factor
IHD	ischaemic heart disease
INR	international normalised ratio
ITU	intensive therapy unit
IUCD	intrauterine contraceptive device
iv	intravenous
IVIG	intravenous immunoglobulin
JVP	jugular venous pressure
LBBB	left bundle-branch block
LDL	low-density lipoprotein
LFTs	liver function tests
LH	luteinising hormone
LMN	lower motor neuron
LMW heparin	low-molecular-weight heparin
LOC	loss of consciousness
LP	lumbar puncture
M3G	morphine-3-glucuronide
M6G	morphine-6-glucuronide
MAO-B	monoamine oxidase B
MCH	mean cell Hb
MCHC	mean cell Hb content
MCL	mid clavicular line
MCV	mean cell volume
MHCT	mental health crisis team
MI	myocardial infarction
MPC	midparental centile
MPH	midparental height
MRA	magnetic resonance angiogram
MRC	Medical Research Council
MRI	magnetic resonance imaging
MST	morphine sulphate tablets
NBM	nil by mouth
NHL	non-Hodgkin's lymphoma

NICE	National Institute for Clinical Excellence
NTD	neural tube defect
OA	osteoarthritis
OCP	oral contraceptive pill
OGTT	oral glucose tolerance test
PA	posteroanterior
PCTA	percutaneous transluminal angioplasty
PCV	packed cell volume
PE	pulmonary embolism
PEA	pulseless electrical activity
POP	progesterone-only pill
prn	as needed
PSA	prostate-specific antigen
PTH	parathyroid hormone
PVD	peripheral vascular disease
qds	four times daily
RA	rheumatoid arthritis
RBCs	red blood cells
RTA	road traffic accident
SAH	subarachnoid haemorrhage
SCT	stem cell transfer
SD	standard deviation
SIADH	syndrome of inappropriate antidiuretic hormone secretion
SIGN	Scottish Intercollegiate Guideline Network
SLE	systemic lupus erythematosus
SOL	space occupying lesion
SSRI	selective serotonin reuptake inhibitor
TAP	typical antipsychotic
TB	tuberculosis
TC	total cholesterol
TCA	tricyclic antidepressant
TCR	target centile range
TIA	transient ischaemic attack
TIBC	total iron-binding capacity
TLE	temporal lobe epilepsy
TSH	thyroid-stimulating hormone
U&Es	urea and electrolytes
UMN	upper motor neuron
USS	ultrasound scan

UTI	urinary tract infection
VC	vomiting centre
VF	ventricular fibrillation
VS	vasovagal syncope
VT	ventricular tachycardia
WBC	white blood cell
WCC	white cell count

SURGICAL CASES:
QUESTIONS

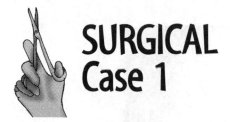

SURGICAL
Case 1

Rachel, a 59-year-old florist, is admitted by her GP to the surgical assessment unit with a history of lower abdominal, colicky pain and increasing constipation for 5 days.

List 2 causes of <u>mechanical</u> large bowel obstruction　　　　　**2 marks**

1.

2.

What signs would you look for in acute <u>mechanical</u> intestinal obstruction?　　　　　**5 marks**

1.

2.

3.

4.

5.

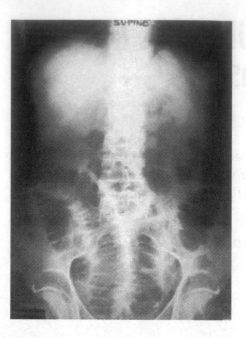

This supine abdominal X-ray (AXR) is from a patient admitted with acute intestinal obstruction.

Is this small or large bowel obstruction? Explain your answer   **2 marks**

1.

2.

On further questioning Rachel admits to having noticed passing some fresh blood mixed with stool on several occasions recently.

List 4 criteria for urgent referral of patients with suspected colorectal cancer   **4 marks**

1.

2.

3.

4.

Rachel undergoes a flexible sigmoidoscopy that detects a lesion in the sigmoid colon. A biopsy is taken and a double-contrast barium enema with bowel preparation (shown below) is subsequently performed.

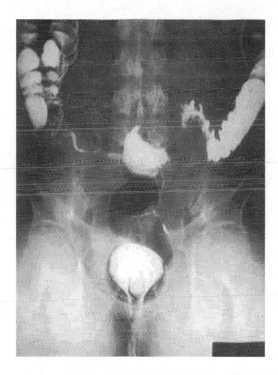

What is the characteristic radiological feature of the lesion in Rachel's sigmoid colon?   ***1 mark***

1.

Rachel undergoes a Hartmann's procedure for her sigmoid cancer with the formation of a stoma in her left iliac fossa. The histopathological findings report that the cancer has extended through the bowel wall, although there is no regional lymph node involvement.

What is the Dukes' classification of Rachel's colon cancer?   ***2 marks***

1.

Name 2 complications of a stoma   *2 marks*

1. _____

2. _____

What member of the community care team should be involved in
Rachel's care?   *2 marks*

1. _____

Total: *20 marks*

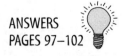

ANSWERS
PAGES 97–102

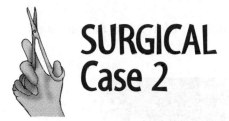 # SURGICAL
Case 2

Ethel, a rather frail 86-year-old who resides at Riverside nursing home, is brought into the emergency department after her carers say that she is 'off her legs' since falling out of bed that morning.

List 6 <u>systemic</u> causes of 'off the legs' in elderly people   ***3 marks***

1. ....

2. ....

3. ....

4. ....

5. ....

6. ....

Your findings on examination of her left leg are consistent with a hip fracture.

What findings would be consistent with a hip fracture?   ***2 marks***

1. ....

2. ....

3. ....

4. ....

You request anteroposterior (AP) (shown below) and lateral X-rays to confirm your diagnosis.

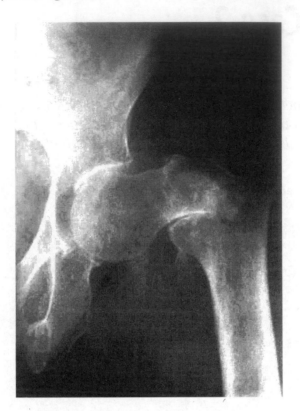

Is this fracture intra- or extracapsular?   **2 marks**

1.

Name a late complication of treating intracapsular fractures by internal fixation as opposed to hemiarthroplasty   **1 mark**

1.

You note, from Ethel's extensive medical history detailed in her accompanying GP notes, that she has several risk factors for a hip fracture, including osteoporosis (for which she is prescribed a bisphosphonate) and a history of falls.

Give 3 pieces of <u>general</u> advice to help prevent osteoporosis   *3 marks*

1.

2.

3.

How do bisphosphonates prevent osteoporosis, what is the main side effect and how is this minimised?   *3 marks*

1.

2.

3.

The orthopaedic surgeon elects to fix Ethel's hip fracture with a dynamic hip screw (DHS) and she is scheduled for surgery the next day.

Ask the FY1 doctor what 8 things should you ensure before surgery?   *4 marks*

1.

2.

3.

4.

5.

6.

7.

8.

Surgery is successful and Ethel is encouraged to start partially weight bearing the following day.

Give 4 reasons why Ethel should start weight bearing asap   **2 marks**

1. _____

2. _____

3. _____

4. _____

Total: **20 marks**

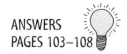

ANSWERS
PAGES 103–108

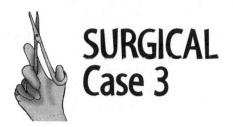

SURGICAL
Case 3

Kristine, a 40-cigarettes-a-day publican, is referred by her GP to the peripheral vascular disease (PVD) clinic with a history of muscular cramp-like pain, mainly in one calf, on walking a short distance, which is rapidly relieved by rest.

What is the differential diagnosis for her leg pain?   **2 marks**

1.

2.

3.

4.

On examination she has absent popliteal and foot pulses in her affected leg.

What non-invasive test confirms the diagnosis of PVD?   **1 mark**

1.

Kristine is discharged back to the care of her GP for treatment of her PVD risk factors.

What are the main <u>modifiable</u> risk factors for PVD?   *2 marks*

1. _____

2. _____

3. _____

4. _____

What advice would you give Kristine?   *3 marks*

1. _____

2. _____

3. _____

Twelve months later Kristine is urgently referred back to the PVD clinic describing a history of deteriorating claudication in the same leg, which has recently progressed to nocturnal rest pain. On examination her affected foot shows signs of critical ischaemia.

What are the signs of a critically ischaemic foot?   *4 marks*

1. _____

2. _____

3. _____

4. _____

Why is pain typically worse at night?   *2 marks*

1. _____

2. _____

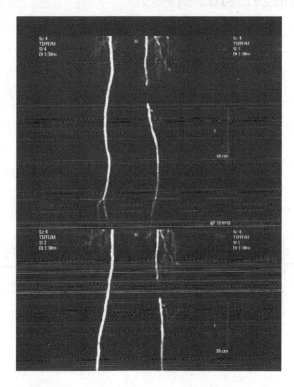

Kristine undergoes a magnetic resonance angiogram (MRA – shown above) and her occluded artery is treated by percutaneous transluminal angioplasty (PTCA).

What artery is occluded?   *2 marks*

1.
_____

Two years later Kristine presents to the emergency department with features of acute limb ischaemia.

List 6 causes of embolic acute lower limb ischaemia   *3 marks*

1.
_____

2.
_____

3. _____

4. _____

5. _____

6. _____

Give 6 features of acute limb ischaemia   *3 marks*

1. _____

2. _____

3. _____

4. _____

5. _____

6. _____

Examination is suggestive of complete acute ischaemia. She is given intravenous heparin and taken straight to theatre for revascularisation of her leg.

Name 3 complications of reperfusion   *3 marks*

1. _____

2. _____

3. _____

Total: *25 marks*

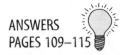

ANSWERS
PAGES 109–115

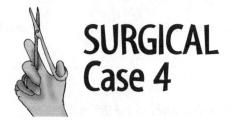

SURGICAL
Case 4

Katie, a 49-year-old art teacher, visits her GP complaining of 'menopausal' symptoms.

What climacteric symptoms may she have?   **2 marks**

1.

2.

3.

4.

She tells you that a friend who is on hormone replacement therapy (HRT) swears by it but is not sure whether it is the best treatment for her.

Of what conditions does HRT increase the risk?   **2 marks**

1.

2.

3.

4.

Which women should receive cyclical progesterone?   *1 mark*

1. _____

It soon becomes obvious that Katie's reluctance for HRT relates to concerns about breast cancer. She wonders why she has not yet been invited for screening.

From what age are women invited to attend the NHS breast-screening programme?   *1 mark*

1. _____

List 6 criteria used in deciding whether to screen for a disease   *3 marks*

1. _____

2. _____

3. _____

4. _____

5. _____

6. _____

She then tells you that this morning she found a lump in her left breast and asks you to examine her for breast cancer.

What signs would you look for on breast examination?   **3 marks**

1.

2.

3.

4.

5.

6.

From the graph below identify which breast lump corresponds to which
peak in incidence   **4 marks**

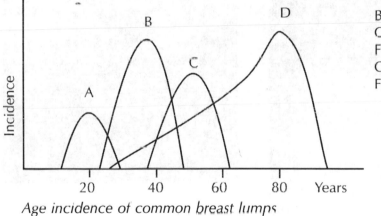

Breast Lump:
Carcinoma
Fibroadenosis
Cyst
Fibroadenoma

Age incidence of common breast lumps

1. A:

2. B:

3. C:

4. D:

On examination you find a lump and, concerned it may be breast cancer, urgently refer her for triple assessment.

What are the 3 components of the triple assessment?   **3 marks**

1. _____

2. _____

3. _____

Katie's mammogram and ultrasound scan (USS) are shown, consistent with breast cancer.

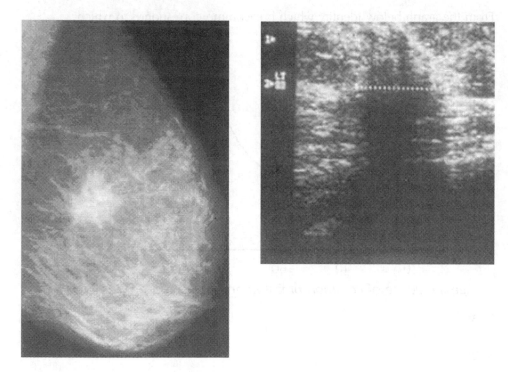

Mammogram (left) demonstrates an irregular mass in the central part of the left breast, which has spicules radiating from it. USS (right) shows a hypoechoic lesion.

Name 4 metastatic sites for breast cancer   **4 marks**

1. ....

2. ....

3. ....

4. ....

List 4 potential treatment options for Katie's breast cancer   **4 marks**

1. ....

2. ....

3. ....

4. ....

What is a sentinel node?   **1 mark**

1. ....

What is the advantage of performing a sentinel node biopsy?   **2 marks**

1. ....

Total: **30 marks**

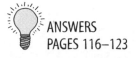
ANSWERS
PAGES 116–123

PSYCHIATRIC CASES: QUESTIONS

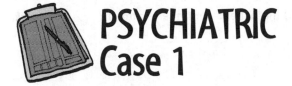

PSYCHIATRIC
Case 1

Lucy visits her GP with symptoms of depression. She has recently separated from her husband and he has moved out of the family home. She tells you she has been feeling down for several months but denies any suicidal thoughts.

Name 8 other symptoms that Lucy may be experiencing **4 marks**

1.

2.

3.

4.

5.

6.

7.

8.

Name a class of antidepressant you would consider prescribing in the first instance: 2 examples and 2 associated side effects **6 marks**

1. Class:

2. Two examples:

3. Two side effects:

For how long after recovery should the patient continue treatment?   *1 mark*

1.

List 2 non-pharmacological treatments of depression   *2 marks*

1.

2.

Several weeks later Lucy presents to the emergency department after taking an overdose of paracetamol. She claims to have taken over 30 tablets (15 g) the night before. A full history, examination and appropriate investigations are taken.

What is considered a potentially fatal dose in adults?   *2 marks*

1.

Outline 10 questions in the history used to assess suicide risk   *5 marks*

1.

2.

3.

4.

5.

6.

7.

8.

9.

10.

Lucy's 11-hour plasma paracetamol concentration is 160 mg/L which is above the normal treatment line shown on the graph.

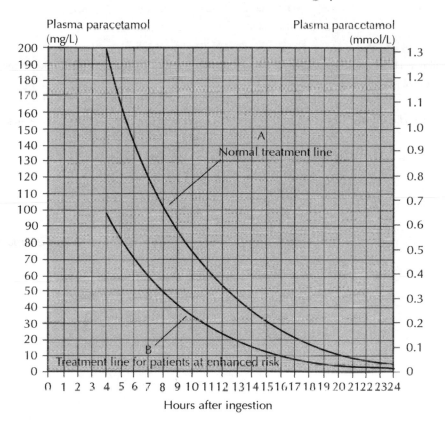

Paracetamol Overdose – Treatment graph

List 2 factors that would put Lucy at enhanced risk **2 marks**

1.

2.

25

What is the antidote for a paracetamol overdose? *1 mark*

1.

Lucy's blood results at the end of the initial antidote treatment are shown below.

Hb	14.1 g/dL	Na+	141 mmol/L	pH	7.37	Bilirubin	16 µmol/L
WCC	8.2 x 10⁹/L	K+	3.9 mmol/L	HCO₃⁻	22 mmol/L	ALT	32 IU/L
Platelets	320 x 10⁹/L	Creatinine	91 µmol/L	P_O	11.4 kPa	ALT	29 IU/L
MCV	85 fL	Urea	4.2 mmol/L	P_{CO_2}	4.9 kPa	ALP	134 IU/L
INR	1.7	Glucose	6.4 mmol/L	BE	-1 mmol/L		

ALP, alkaline phosphatase; ALT, alanine transaminase; BE base excess; Hb, haemoglobin; INR, international normalised ratio; MCV, mean cell volume; WCC, white cell count.

Is she <u>medically</u> fit for discharge; justify your answer? *2 marks*

1.

2.

Total: *25 marks*

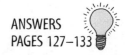

ANSWERS
PAGES 127–133

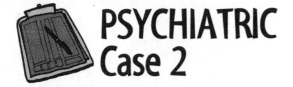

PSYCHIATRIC
Case 2

Sarah is a 21-year-old college student still living at home. Her mother calls out the GP, concerned that Sarah seems to have become very withdrawn, hardly ever leaving her room and refusing to let her in. She has also started wearing a hat made of kitchen foil 'to stop them from hearing what I'm thinking'.

What is a hallucination?   **2 marks**

1.

From what psychotic symptom is Sarah suffering?   **1 mark**

1.

The GP, concerned that Sarah's health is at risk, tries to persuade her to come into hospital for further assessment.

What Act may be used to compulsorily treat psychiatric patients?   **2 marks**

1.

How long can patients be detained under Section 2 of this Act?   **1 mark**

1.

Sarah is admitted to the psychiatric hospital where she is subsequently diagnosed with schizophrenia.

What is the differential diagnosis?   *3 marks*

1.

2.

3.

List 4 first-rank symptoms of schizophrenia   *4 marks*

1.

2.

3.

4.

Sarah's psychiatrist prescribes an antipsychotic.

What is the mechanism of action of <u>typical</u> antipsychotics?   *1 mark*

1.

List 4 extrapyramidal symptoms (EPSs) of antipsychotics   *4 marks*

1.

2.

3.

4.

What type of drug is used to treat EPSs?   *1 mark*

1.

_____

*Sarah's symptoms are unresponsive to several antipsychotics, so
eventually she is started on clozapine.*

What weekly test will Sarah need?   *1 mark*

1.

_____

Total: **20 marks**

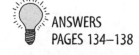

ANSWERS
PAGES 134–138

29

HAEMATOLOGY CASES:
QUESTIONS

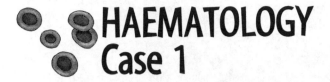

HAEMATOLOGY
Case 1

After a routine blood test that reported lymphocytosis, Andrew, a 54-year-old advertising executive, is recalled by his GP. On examination the only finding of note is cervical lymphadenopathy; he is otherwise asymptomatic.

List 4 causes of lymphadenopathy   ***4 marks***

1.

2.

3.

4.

Andrew is referred to the haematology outpatient clinic where he is diagnosed with chronic lymphocytic leukaemia (CLL). As a result of the early stage of his disease he is simply monitored; within 24 months he is symptomatic, has moderate splenomegaly and is anaemic.

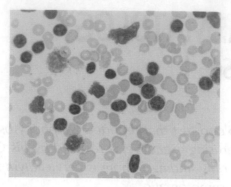

Andrew's peripheral blood film showing stained lymphocytes with thin rims of cytoplasm, coarse condensed nuclear chromatin and characteristic smear (or smudge) cells.

Name 4 causes of splenomegaly   **4 marks**

1.

2.

3.

4.

Give 4 reasons why CLL patients may be anaemic   **4 marks**

1.

2.

3.

4.

As a result of the progressive nature of his disease, Andrew's haematologist starts him on cytotoxic chemotherapy with fludarabine.

Haematology

Name 6 side effects of cytotoxic chemotherapy   **3 marks**

1.

2.

3.

4.

5.

6.

What drug is used to prevent tumour lysis syndrome?   **1 mark**

1.

After chemotherapy Andrew goes into complete remission (CR). He is entered into the MRC CLL5 trial comparing 'autologous stem cell transfer (SCT) against no treatment following first-line chemotherapy'.

List 6 points you need to inform patients of when entering them into a clinical trial   **6 marks**

1.

2.

3.

4.

5.

6.

Against which opportunistic infection are SCT patients given prophylactic co-trimoxazole (Septrin)? **1 mark**

1.

Give 1 advantage and 1 disadvantage of autologous (self) over allogeneic (donor) SCT **2 marks**

Advantage:

1.

Disadvantage:

1.

Total: **25 marks**

ANSWERS
PAGES 141–146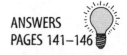

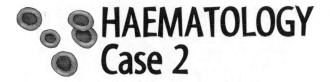

HAEMATOLOGY
Case 2

Lisa, a 22-year-old charity administrator, visits her GP with a 9-month history of progressive fatigue that has become more marked recently. On examination she is clinically anaemic.

Of what other anaemic symptoms may she be complaining?   **2 marks**

1.

2.

3.

4.

The GP requests a full blood count (FBC), reticulocyte count, iron studies, vitamin B_{12} and folate levels, and a peripheral blood film.

FBC	Lisa's results	Normal range (female)
Hb (g/dL)	8.8	11.5–16
MCV (fL)	73	76–96
PCV (haematocrit) (%)	27.4	37–47
MCH (pg)	23.3	27–32
MCHC (g/dL)	31.9	30–36
WCC (x10⁹/L)	5.2	4–11
Platelets (x10⁹/L)	243	150–400

FBC, full blood count; Hb, haemoglobin; MCH, mean cell Hb; MCHC, mean cell Hb content; PCV, packed cell volume; WCC, white cell count.

Name 3 causes of microcytic (low MCV) anaemia **3 marks**

1.

2.

3.

Name 3 causes of macrocytic (high MCV) anaemia **3 marks**

1.

2.

3.

In iron-deficiency anaemia and anaemia of chronic disease indicate
(↑↔↓) at ? the expected changes **3 marks**

	Iron-deficiency anaemia	Anaemia of chronic disease	Normal range (females)
Serum ferritin (µg/L)	?	?	14–150
Serum iron (µmol/L)	?	?	10–30
TIBC (µmol/L)	?	?	40–75
(TIBC, total iron-binding capacity.)			

Lisa's iron studies indicate that she is iron deficient. She denies menorrhagia and claims to eat a healthy, balanced diet. Her vitamin B_{12} and folate levels and reticulocyte count are shown below.

	Lisa's results	Normal range (females)
Reticulocyte count (x10^9/L)	32	25–100
Serum vitamin B_{12} (ng/L)	280	160–925
Serum folate (µg/L)	1.9	2.8–13.5

Haematology

What test is used to distinguish between vitamin B_{12} deficiency caused by malabsorption and lack of intrinsic factor (IF)? **1 mark**

1.

Briefly describe what this test involves **1 mark**

1.

On further questioning she admits that she has lost weight and passes frequent loose stools. Suspecting malabsorption as the cause of her iron and folate deficiency anaemia, Lisa is subsequently diagnosed with coeliac disease.

List 4 other causes of malabsorption **4 marks**

1.

2.

3.

4.

What other condition is associated with folate deficiency? **1 mark**

1.

Lisa is placed on a gluten-free diet and given iron and folate supplements for 6 months, during which time her blood counts recover.

Haematology

List 2 side effects of oral iron about which you should warn Lisa   *1 mark*

1.

2.

Name 2 other long-term complications of coeliac disease   *1 mark*

1.

2.

Total: *20 marks*

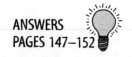

ANSWERS
PAGES 147–152

ENDOCRINOLOGY CASES:
QUESTIONS

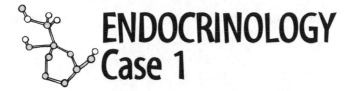

ENDOCRINOLOGY
Case 1

Andy, a 47-year-old estate agent, visits his GP complaining of general tiredness. He's a non-smoker but admits to eating and drinking to excess. On examination he weighs 95 kg and his height is 1.72 m; his BP is 154/92 mmHg.

Calculate his body mass index (BMI) **1 mark**

1.

His urine dipstick is ++ for glucose.

How would you confirm the diagnosis of diabetes? **2 marks**

1.

2.

List 4 other presenting symptoms of type 2 diabetes **4 marks**

1.

2.

3.

4.

Initially Andy attempts to manage his diabetes mellitus by diet and exercise alone, but this fails to control his hyperglycaemia.

On what hypoglycaemic agent would you start Andy?   *1 mark*

1.

Andy is reviewed 6 monthly to monitor his glycaemic control and assess the development of any diabetic complications.

How do you assess long-term glycaemic control?   *1 mark*

1.

Andy's fasting lipids are measured: total cholesterol (TC) 6.34 mmol/L, low-density lipoprotein (LDL) 4.22 mmol/L, high-density lipoprotein (HDL) 1.26 mmol/L, triglycerides 2.4 mmol/L.

Calculate his 10-year coronary heart disease (CHD) risk   *2 marks*

1.

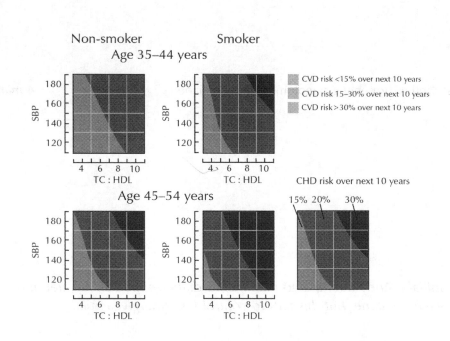

How do you screen for diabetic renal disease?   **2 marks**

1.
....

2.
....

What is the first-line treatment of hypertension in the presence of diabetic renal disease?   **1 mark**

1.
....

Andy's feet are examined: he has bilateral foot pulses but is unable to perceive the pressure from a 10 g monofilament and so is at increased risk of developing a 'diabetic foot'.

List 4 pieces of preventive foot care advice   **4 marks**

1.
....

2.
....

3.
....

4.
....

As part of his diabetes review, Andy also attends the local optometrist (report as follows): bilateral microaneurysms and microhaemorrhages present, extensive hard exudates noted. No cotton-wool spots detected. No new vessel formation. Visual acuity (while wearing spectacles): 6/6 (left), 6/6 (right).

Classify Andy's diabetic retinopathy   **2 marks**

1.
....

ANSWERS
PAGES 155–160

Total: **20 marks**

Endocrinology

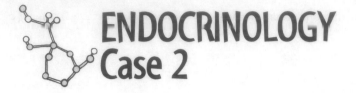

ENDOCRINOLOGY
Case 2

As the surgical FY1 on call you are bleeped to see Zoe, an orthopaedic patient, 2 days after a total hip replacement, with the biochemical results shown below.

	Zoe's results	Normal range
Na+ (mmol/L)	124	135–145
K+ (mmol/L)	4.3	3.5–5
Urea (mmol/L)	3.2	2.5–6.7
Creatinine (µmol/L)	88	70–150
Albumin (g/L)	37	35–50
Glucose (mmol/L)	5.2	4–6

Give 2 common causes of iatrogenic hyponatraemia on the wards   **2 marks**

1.

2.

One of the medical students on your ward suggests giving Zoe hypertonic intravenous saline to correct her low Na+.

Give 2 clinical features of <u>severe</u> hyponatraemia   **2 marks**

1.

2.

Would you give Zoe hypertonic saline? What is the main risk?   **2 marks**

1.

2.

You assess Zoe to determine whether she is dehydrated or fluid overloaded.

How would you assess Zoe's fluid balance?   **4 marks**

1.

2.

3.

4.

Name 4 causes of hyponatraemia in fluid-overloaded patients   **2 marks**

1.

2.

3.

4.

How would you manage hyponatraemia in such patients?   **1 mark**

1.

How would you exclude renal Na$^+$ loss in dehydrated patients?   **1 mark**

1.

What other electrolyte abnormality would you expect in Addison's disease?   **1 mark**

1.

Zoe is neither dehydrated nor fluid overloaded so you request a urinary Na⁺ and osmolality, which are reported as 32 mmol/L and 400 mosmol/L, respectively.

Calculate Zoe's plasma osmolality   *2 marks*

1.

What is the likely cause of her hyponatraemia?   *1 mark*

1.

How could you treat her hyponatraemia?   *2 marks*

1.

2.

Total: *20 marks*

ANSWERS
PAGES 161–165

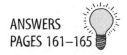

Endocrinology

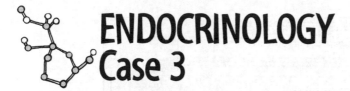

ENDOCRINOLOGY
Case 3

Jack, aged 15, is concerned about his height. He is the shortest in his class and although he enjoys football he finds that he can't keep up with the much bigger boys in his year. His parents, worried about his growth, have taken regular measurements of his height over the past 5 years, as shown below.

Age (years)	Height (cm)	Age (years)	Height (cm)
10	134	13	145
11	138	14	147
12	142	15	149

His parents are of average height: his dad is 172 cm and his mum is 164 cm.

Plot Jack's height measurements on the growth chart.   **3 marks**

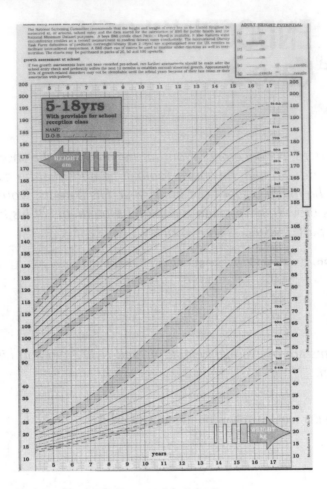

Why is it important to know the parents' heights? *2 marks*

1.

_____

Apart from being small, Jack also seems to be a slow developer. A lot of his friends are already shaving and their voices have broken, whereas Jack has no pubertal features yet.

Describe the hormone axis that regulates puberty *2 marks*

1.

_____

What is the first sign of puberty in boys?   *2 marks*

1.

What is the name of the puberty staging system?   *1 mark*

1.

What non-invasive investigation can be used to assess growth in Jack?   *1 mark*

1.

Which diagnosis is important to exclude in short females with no signs
of puberty?   *2 marks*

1.

What is the most likely cause of Jack's short stature?   *2 marks*

1.

Give 5 other causes of short stature   *5 marks*

1.

2.

3.

4.

5.

ANSWERS
PAGES 166–170

Total: *20 marks*

EMERGENCY MEDICINE CASES: QUESTIONS

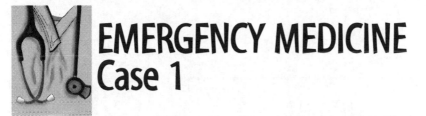

EMERGENCY MEDICINE
Case 1

Gary, a 23-year-old man, is brought into the emergency department after a high-speed road traffic accident (RTA). He has sustained trauma to the left side of his head and has a reduced level of consciousness.

List 3 causes of secondary brain injury **3 marks**

1.

2.

3.

Gary's neck is immobilised, his ABCs are stabilised and an assessment of his neurological status undertaken. His Glasgow Coma Score (GCS) is assessed as follows: his eyes open to pain, he localises pain and his speech is confused.

Calculate Gary's GCS **2 marks**

1.

A full examination reveals that Gary has sustained no other major injuries.

List 4 signs on examination of a basal skull fracture **2 marks**

1.

2.

55

3. _____

4. _____

Other than ↓GCS list 6 other criteria under which you would admit a
patient after a head injury   *3 marks*

1. _____

2. _____

3. _____

4. _____

5. _____

6. _____

List 6 regular observations that Gary should undergo   *6 marks*

1. _____

2. _____

3. _____

4. _____

5. _____

6. _____

Emergency Medicine

*Gary's GCS continues to deteriorate so he undergoes an urgent
computed tomography (CT) scan of his head.*

Describe 2 abnormalities seen on his CT scan   *2 marks*

1. _____

2. _____

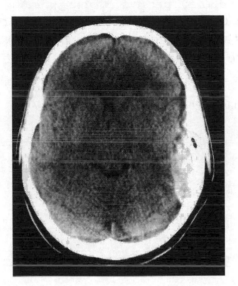

Gary's brain CT scan.

What is the diagnosis?   *1 mark*

1. _____

What further course of action should be undertaken?   *1 mark*

1. _____

Total: *20 marks*

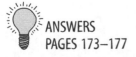
ANSWERS
PAGES 173–177

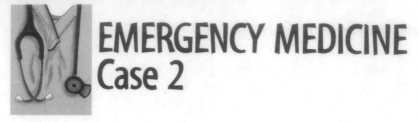

EMERGENCY MEDICINE
Case 2

Rob, a 26-year-old PE teacher, is refereeing a game of football when he complains of a severe occipital headache before vomiting and collapsing on the playing field.

What is the differential diagnosis of a severe headache?   **2 marks**

1.

2.

3.

4.

Rob is rushed to the emergency department where on admittance his GCS is 7.

List 6 causes of coma   **3 marks**

1.

2.

3.

4.

5.

6.

An emergency brain CT can is performed which shows blood within the basal cisterns (subarachnoid reservoirs at the base of the brain containing large pools of cerebrospinal fluid [CSF]) of Rob's brain, confirming the diagnosis of a subarachnoid haemorrhage (SAH).

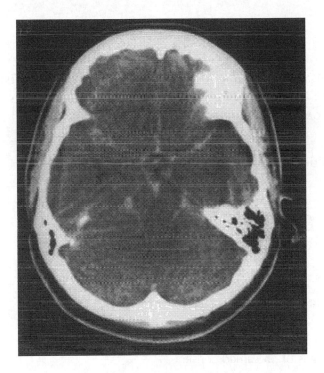

If Rob's CT was negative how would you exclude an SAH?   **2 marks**

1.

___

How do you prevent vasospasm after a bleed?   **1 mark**

1.

___

Rob is transferred to the intensive therapy unit (ITU) but as a result of the severity of his bleed continues to deteriorate. Several days later he is diagnosed as 'brain dead'.

Describe 4 of the tests used to diagnose brain-stem death   **4 marks**

Emergency Medicine

1.
_____

2.
_____

3.
_____

4.
_____

Rob is considered suitable for organ donation so his girlfriend and parents are approached for permission, because his wishes regarding organ donation are unknown.

List 4 patient criteria for organ donation   **2 marks**

1.
_____

2.
_____

3.
_____

4.
_____

Give 3 advantages of presumed consent   **3 marks**

1.
_____

2.
_____

3.
_____

List 3 acceptable and 3 unacceptable criteria for receiving a transplant   **3 marks**

Acceptable:

1.

2.

3.

Unacceptable:

1.

2.

3.

Total: **20 marks**

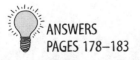

ANSWERS
PAGES 178–183

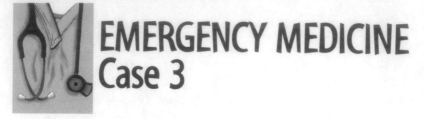

EMERGENCY MEDICINE
Case 3

Simon, a 69-year-old known patient with ischaemic heart disease (IHD), is brought into the emergency department with several hours' history of progressive shortness of breath.

What is the differential diagnosis? **2 marks**

1.

2.

3.

4.

On examination he is clearly distressed, sweaty and pale, with signs consistent with acute heart failure.

What are the signs of acute <u>left ventricular failure?</u> **3 marks**

1.

2.

3.

4.

5.

6.

What is your immediate management? **2 marks**

1.

2.

3. _____

4. _____

You request a CXR and ECG, and take bloods for FBC, urea and electrolytes (U&Es), troponin T and arterial blood gases (ABGs).

Parameter	Simon's results	Normal range
pH	7.24	7.35–7.45
PO_2 (kPa)	11.8 (on 100% O_2)	> 10.6
PCO_2 (kPa)	6.94	7–6
HCO_3^- (mmol/L)	14.6	24–30
BE	-11.2	± 2

What do these ABG results indicate?   *1 mark*

1. _____

Simon's erect AP CXR is shown.

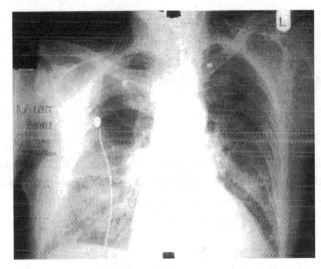

Identify 3 abnormalities on his CXR   *3 marks*

1. _____

2. _____

3. _____

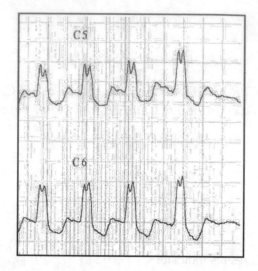

Simon's ECG (leads V5–6) is shown in the figure.

What does his ECG show?   **1 mark**

1.

How would you confirm that this is a new ECG change?   **1 mark**

1.

Simon is transferred to the coronary care unit (CCU) for continuous ECG monitoring. Later that night he arrests in asystole. The nurse on duty dials 2222 to summon the cardiac arrest team and commences basic life support (BLS).

List 3 other rhythms associated with cardiac arrest   **3 marks**

1.

2.

3.

How would you manage the arrest? **3 marks**

1.

2.

3.

List 8 potential reversible causes of cardiac arrest **4 marks**

1.

2.

3.

4.

5.

6.

7.

8.

Give 4 situations where CPR (cardiopulmonary resuscitation) should not
be attempted **2 marks**

1.

2.

3.

4.

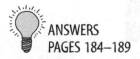 ANSWERS
PAGES 184–189

Total: **25 marks**

65

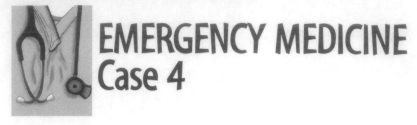

EMERGENCY MEDICINE
Case 4

Dan, an otherwise healthy 22-year-old student, is admitted to the emergency department with sudden onset of right-sided pleuritic chest pain and breathlessness.

What is the differential diagnosis?   **4 marks**

1. _____

2. _____

3. _____

4. _____

Indicate (↑↔↓) the expected findings consistent with a pneumothorax   **3 marks**

Findings on the affected side

Breath sounds   ?

Chest wall expansion   ?

Percussion note   ?

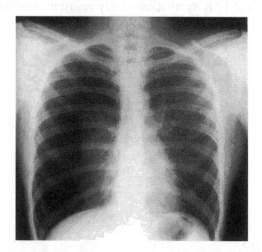

A CXR is ordered which shows a large right-sided pneumothorax.

What radiological and clinical features would indicate a <u>tension</u>
pneumothorax?   *2 marks*

Radiological:

1.
_____

Clinical:

1.
_____

What action should be taken in Dan's case?   *1 mark*

1.
_____

Assuming his weight is 70 kg, what volume of 1% lidocaine can be safely
administered (maximum dose 3 mg/kg)   *2 marks*

1.
_____

*The chest X-ray is repeated showing only a slight improvement in
the pneumothorax with no improvement in Dan's symptoms.*

What further action could be taken?   *2 marks*

1.
_____

2.
_____

A 12-gauge Seldinger chest drain is inserted into the right fifth intercostal space (ICS) anterior to the midaxillary line and attached to an underwater seal. A repeat CXR 24 hours later shows expansion of the right lung field, although the pneumothorax is still present.

What action should be taken next?   *1 mark*

1.

Should the drain be clamped before removal?   *1 mark*

1.

What advice should be given to Dan before discharge?   *2 marks*

1.

2.

This is Dan's second right-sided pneumothorax.

What further treatment should be advised?   *2 marks*

1.

2.

Total: *20 marks*

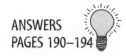

ANSWERS
PAGES 190–194

NEUROLOGICAL CASES: QUESTIONS

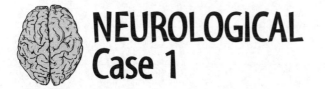

NEUROLOGICAL
Case 1

Mark, a 73-year-old widower, is referred to the emergency outpatient department by his GP with a 12-month history of progressive difficulty in walking and recurrent falls.

List 6 possible causes of falls in elderly people   **6 marks**

1.

2.

3.

4.

5.

6.

As Mark enters the consultation room you note that he has a very slow, shuffling gait suggestive of Parkinson's disease.

What are the 3 main features of Parkinson's disease?   **3 marks**

1.

2.

3.

List 3 differentiating features of a parkinsonian tremor   **3 marks**

1. _____

2. _____

3. _____

On the basis of the history and examination you confirm a diagnosis of Parkinson's disease.

Other than Parkinson's disease, list 2 other causes of parkinsonism   ***2 marks***

1. _____

2. _____

What is the underlying pathophysiology of Parkinson's disease?   ***2 marks***

1. _____

Several months later Mark is started on L-dopa, which greatly improves his parkinsonian symptoms.

What class of drug is combined with L-dopa to prevent peripheral side effects?   ***1 mark***

1. _____

Name 3 complications of L-dopa therapy   ***3 marks***

1. _____

2. _____

3. _____

Total: ***20 marks***

ANSWERS
PAGES 197–201

Neurological

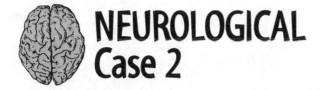

NEUROLOGICAL
Case 2

Jo, a 21-year-old student, is brought into the emergency department after having blacked out while watching TV at home with one of her flatmates.

Give 4 causes of <u>syncope</u>   **2 marks**

1. _____

2. _____

3. _____

4. _____

What 6 questions would you ask Jo's flatmate <u>about the attack itself?</u>   **6 marks**

1. _____

2. _____

3. _____

4. _____

5. _____

6. _____

Jo's flatmate tells you that Jo suddenly stopped talking, fell to the floor and then started moving her arms and legs in jerky movements. Jo has no memory of the attack itself but says that she had no warning of it happening.

List 6 causes of seizures   *3 marks*

1.

2.

3.

4.

5.

6.

What type of seizure did Jo have?   *1 mark*

1.

Give 4 features of temporal lobe epilepsy (TLE)   *2 marks*

1.

2.

3.

4.

What is the most useful investigation to confirm the diagnosis of
epilepsy?   *1 mark*

1.

*Several weeks later Jo has a second seizure and the neurologist
decides to start her on anticonvulsive treatment.*

Neurological

What is first-line treatment for Jo's type of seizure?   *2 marks*

1.
———

What advice do you give women of childbearing age about antiepileptic drugs?   *3 marks*

1.
———

2.
———

3.
———

Total: *20 marks*

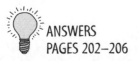

ANSWERS
PAGES 202–206

PALLIATIVE CARE CASES:
QUESTIONS

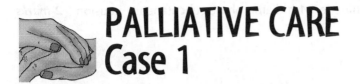

PALLIATIVE CARE
Case 1

Julia has breast cancer with bone metastases. She has had two recent hospital admissions for hypercalcaemia and is now on monthly pamidronate infusions. She takes diclofenac 75 mg twice daily (bd) and morphine sulphate tablets (MST) 120 mg bd for bone pain.

Describe the 3 steps of the analgesic ladder   **3 marks**

1. Step 1:

2. Step 2:

3. Step 3:

List 4 side effects of morphine   **4 marks**

1.

2.

3.

4.

Why should morphine be used with caution in renal failure?   **1 mark**

1.

Unfortunately, her condition has deteriorated rapidly over the last week and she is admitted to St John's Hospice. She is nauseous with occasional vomiting, in obvious pain and unable to take oral medications.

Convert her oral morphine to 24-h diamorphine subcutaneous infusion **2 marks**

1.

Give 4 potential causes of Julia's nausea and vomiting **4 marks**

1.

2.

3.

4.

Julia is prescribed metoclopramide for her nausea and vomiting.

Where does metoclopramide exert its antiemetic effect? **1 mark**

1.

It is clear that Julia is terminally ill and it is decided to no longer treat her hypercalcaemia.

List 4 factors that need to be considered when deciding to withdraw treatment **2 marks**

1.

2.

3.

4.

Despite the analgesia Julia still continues to experience breakthrough pain. The nurse is reluctant to prescribe diamorphine as needed (prn) for fear of hastening Julia's death.

Give 3 reasons why such treatment is not considered to be euthanasia   **3 marks**

1. ....

2. ....

3. ....

Total: **20 marks**

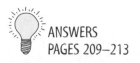
ANSWERS
PAGES 209–213

Palliative Care

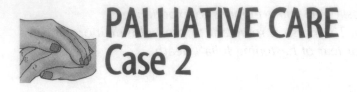

PALLIATIVE CARE
Case 2

Michael, a 72-year-old farmer, visits his GP complaining of several months' history of worsening back pain which is now no longer eased by paracetamol.

List 4 sinister back pain symptoms   **4 marks**

1.

2.

3.

4.

Name 4 primary cancers that metastasise to bone   **2 marks**

1.

2.

3.

4.

The GP requests a number of outpatient investigations as below.

Palliative Care

Investigation	Michael's result	Normal range	Investigation	Michael's result	Normal range
Hb (g/dL)	11.2	13–18	Na⁺ (mmol/L)	142	135–145
MCV (fL)	91	76–96	K⁺ (mmol/L)	4.1	3.5–5
WCC (x10⁹/L)	7	4–11	Urea (mmol/L)	6.6	2.5–6.7
Platelets (x10⁹/L)	220	150–400	Creatinine (µmol/L)	138	70–150
ESR (mm/h)	89	<30	Ca²⁺ (mmol/L)	2.7	2.12–2.65
			Proteins (g/L)	72	60–80
Urine dipstick	Protein	+++	Albumin (g/L)	25	35–50
Spinal X-ray	No vertebral fracture		ALP (IU/L)	70	30–150
PSA (µg/L)	3.4	<4			

ALP, alkaline phosphatase; ALT, alanine transaminase; ESR, erythrocyte sedimentation rate; Hb, haemoglobin; MCV, mean cell volume; PSA, prostate-specific antigen; WCC, white cell count.

Suspecting that myeloma is the cause of his back pain, Michael's GP refers him to the haematologists where the diagnosis is confirmed.

List 2 myeloma diagnostic criteria   **2 marks**

1.

2.

What does his lateral skull X-ray show?   **1 mark**

1. _____

Michael is treated with melphalan (for his myeloma) and a bisphosphonate (for his bone disease).

Calculate Michael's adjusted Ca^{2+} ***1 mark***

1. _____

Give 4 symptoms of hypercalcaemia   ***4 marks***

1. _____

2. _____

3. _____

4. _____

Michael's myeloma enters into remission, his melphalan is stopped and he is monitored as an outpatient. Some 18 months later his myeloma relapses and he is admitted with suspected cord compression confirmed by MRI.

List 4 other causes of cord <u>compression</u>   ***4 marks***

1. _____

2. _____

3. _____

4. _____

Palliative Care

Name 4 <u>motor</u> signs you would expect to find <u>below</u> the site of a cord lesion **4 marks**

1.

2.

3.

4.

Total: **20 marks**

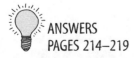
ANSWERS
PAGES 214–219

PAEDIATRIC CASES:
QUESTIONS

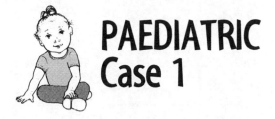

PAEDIATRIC
Case 1

Sam, a 2-year-old boy of African-Caribbean descent, is referred to Alder Hey after his mother has noticed that his fingers seem swollen and that he always seems tired. He is subsequently diagnosed with sickle-cell disease (SCD).

What is the inheritance of sickle-cell disease? **1 mark**

1.

What is the pathogenesis of sickle-cell anaemia? **2 marks**

1.

2.

Sam's mum is very upset about the diagnosis and worries that any future children will also be affected.

To where should mum be referred? **1 mark**

1.

Sam's mother is told that sickle-cell disease cannot be prevented but that it is possible to screen for it during pregnancy.

Give 2 advantages and 2 disadvantages of antenatal screening **4 marks**

Advantages:

1.

2.

Disadvantages:

1.

2.

Now aged 4, Sam presents with a painful left hip and a temperature of 38.5°C. He refuses to weight bear on his left leg and mum denies a history of trauma.

Give 2 differential diagnoses   ***2 marks***

1.

2.

List 4 factors that may precipitate a crisis   ***2 marks***

1.

2.

3.

4.

Give 4 prophylactic measures important for SCD patients   ***4 marks***

1.

2.

3. ....

4. ....

Now aged 9, Sam's condition has markedly deteriorated as a result of numerous, severe crises and it is now decided that he should have regular blood transfusions.

Give 4 <u>acute</u> complications of blood transfusions   **4 marks**

1. ....

2. ....

3. ....

4. ....

Give 5 <u>long-term</u> complications of SCD   **5 marks**

1. ....

2. ....

3. ....

4. ....

5. ....

Total: **25 marks**

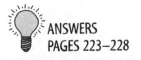
ANSWERS
PAGES 223–228

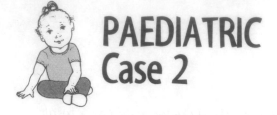

PAEDIATRIC
Case 2

Charlie is a 1-year-old, happy and thriving little girl. However, mum attends the community health centre because she is a bit worried that Charlie is a bit 'behind' all her friends. The health visitor carries out a development screening test noting the following:

Gross motor: Good head control, sits with support but not by herself, hasn't started crawling yet

Fine motor and vision: Follows an object, reaches out to grasp, transfers toys with right hand to mouth, points with right index finger and has a good palmar grasp. During the test she doesn't use her left hand, which is kept closed

Hearing and speech: Turns to sound of name, vocalises when she is on her own, uses mummy and daddy and can say two to three more words

Social behaviour and play: She smiles, puts everything into her mouth, waves bye-bye and tries drinking from a cup

What are the worrying features in this assessment?   **3 marks**

1.

2.

3.

As part of her assessment the health visitor also checks Charlie's immunisation status.

What immunisations should Charlie have had and when?   **3 marks**

1.
....

2.
....

The health visitor is worried that Charlie may have cerebral palsy.

Name 6 other clinical features of cerebral palsy   **6 marks**

1.
....

2.
....

3.
....

4.
....

5.
....

6.
....

List 6 causes of cerebral palsy   **3 marks**

1.
....

2.
....

3.
....

4.
....

5.
....

6.
....

Over the next year Charlie starts to walk but Mum notices that her left leg is stiff, and when she walks she walks on tiptoes because she can't put her left foot flat on the floor.

What clinical type of cerebral palsy has Charlie developed?   **2 marks**

1.

_____

What other features of this motor pattern may you find on examining her left leg?   **4 marks**

1.

_____

2.

_____

3.

_____

4.

_____

Charlie is referred to the child development service for assessment and management of her cerebral palsy.

List 4 members of the child development team   **4 marks**

1.

_____

2.

_____

3.

_____

4.

_____

Total: **25 marks**

ANSWERS
PAGES 229–233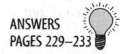

SURGICAL CASES:
ANSWERS

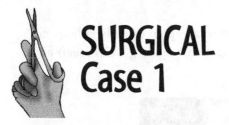

SURGICAL
Case 1

*Rachel, a 59-year-old florist, is admitted by her GP to the surgical
assessment unit with a history of lower abdominal, colicky pain and
increasing constipation for 5 days.*

List 2 causes of <u>mechanical</u> large bowel obstruction   ***2 marks***

**Intestinal obstruction is either functional (ie lumen not blocked but reduced
bowel motility, eg after surgery, peritonitis) or mechanical (ie blocked lumen):**

1. Colorectal cancer.

2. Volvulus (twisting of loop of bowel).

🌑 Causes of small bowel obstruction include adhesions (eg after previous
surgery), hernias, gallstone ileus, ingested foreign body and strictures
(eg Crohn's disease).

What signs would you look for in acute <u>mechanical</u> intestinal
obstruction?   ***5 marks***

1. Abdominal distension.

**2. Abdominal tenderness (in strangulated bowel, eg volvulus, you may get
peritonism with raised white cell count [WCC], pulse and temperature).**

3. Visible peristalsis.

4. Hernias: check both inguinal and femoral sites.

5. Rectal mass on per rectum (PR) examination.

6. Increased (tinkling) bowel sounds (absent in paralytic ileus).

QUESTIONS
PAGES 3–6

ⓘ The four cardinal symptoms of obstruction are: pain (usually colicky but may be constant if strangulated), constipation, vomiting (with relief) and distension.

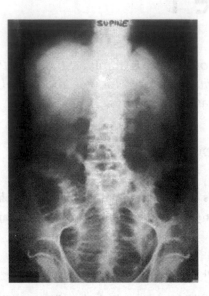

This supine abdominal X-ray (AXR) is from a patient admitted with acute intestinal obstruction.

Is this small or large bowel obstruction? Explain your answer   *2 marks*

1. Small bowel obstruction.

2. Circular folds cross the full width of the lumen of the distended loops, indicating that this is small bowel.

ⓘ Abdominal X-ray is primarily used to investigate the acute abdomen (also erect chest X-ray [CXR] to exclude air under the diaphragm). The small bowel is recognised by circular folds (plicae circulares) that cross the full width of the bowel lumen (they also tend to be more central); in the large bowel the haustral folds go only part way across the lumen (and tend to be more peripheral). In obstruction, look for abnormal gas patterns (when supine) and dilated bowel (abnormal if small bowel > 3 cm and large bowel > 6 cm).

🔵 Never let the 'sun go up and down' on acute obstruction because the risk of complications, eg perforation, from delayed intervention is high.

On further questioning Rachel admits to having noticed passing some fresh blood mixed with stool on several occasions recently.

List 4 criteria for urgent referral of patients with suspected colorectal cancer **4 marks**

1. **Increased frequency of defecation or looser stools (≥6 weeks).**

2. **Rectal bleeding.**

3. **Iron-deficient anaemia without an obvious cause.**

4. **Palpable rectal mass.**

5. **Palpable abdominal mass.**

🔵 The referral guidelines of the National Institute for Clinical Excellence (NICE) are:

(a) **Rectal bleeding <u>with</u> a change in bowel habit to looser stools and/or <u>increased</u> frequency of defecation ≥6 weeks in <u>all</u> ages (decreased frequency of defecation is low risk for cancer).**

(b) **Change in bowel habit to looser stools and/or increased frequency of defecation ≥6 weeks <u>without</u> rectal bleeding in those aged > 60 years.**

(c) **A definite, palpable, right-sided, abdominal mass in <u>all</u> ages.**

(d) **A definite, palpable, rectal (not pelvic) mass in <u>all</u> ages.**

(e) **Rectal bleeding <u>without</u> anal symptoms (eg soreness, itching) in those aged > 60 years.**

(f) **Iron-deficient anaemia without an obvious cause, eg menstruation, in <u>all</u> ages.**

🔵 About 80% of patients with colorectal cancer present with these symptoms and should be urgently referred (with <2-week wait) for further investigation. Twenty per cent of patients at presentation are admitted as surgical emergencies, eg large bowel obstruction, abdominal pain.

Rachel undergoes a flexible sigmoidoscopy that detects a lesion in the sigmoid colon. A biopsy is taken and a double-contrast barium enema with bowel preparation (shown below) is subsequently performed.

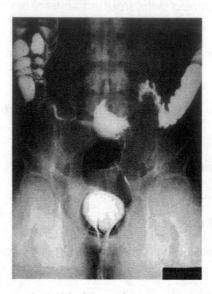

What is the characteristic radiological feature of the lesion in Rachel's sigmoid colon?

1 mark

1. Apple-core lesion: this is the typical appearance of colon cancer.

🟦 Colorectal cancer can usually be visualised by endoscopy (either colonoscopy or sigmoidoscopy). About 70% of colorectal cancer occur in the rectosigmoid area where they can be visualised by flexible sigmoidoscopy (which can reach the splenic flexure).

🟦 The initial investigation in colorectal cancer is flexible sigmoidoscopy (colonoscopy if symptoms suggest cancer of right side or transverse colon, eg iron-deficiency anaemia). Barium enemas are very effective at imaging structural abnormalities and are commonly used by surgeons in planning surgical intervention (although in some hospitals it is being replaced by computed tomography [CT] colonography).

Rachel undergoes a Hartmann's procedure for her sigmoid cancer with the formation of a stoma in her left iliac fossa. The histopathological findings report that the cancer has extended through the bowel wall, although there is no regional lymph node involvement.

What is the Dukes' classification of Rachel's colon cancer?   ***2 marks***

1. Dukes' B.

Colorectal cancer is classified as follows:

Dukes' A: confined to bowel wall – 90% 5-year survival rate.

Dukes' B: extension through bowel wall – 75% 5-year survival rate.

Dukes' C: involvement of regional lymph nodes – 30% 5-year survival rate.

Dukes' D: distant metastases (typically the liver) – <5% 5-year survival rate.

Surgical resection is the most effective curative treatment (palliative for Dukes' D). The procedure depends on the site, eg hemicolectomy with end-to-end anastomosis for ascending, transverse and descending colonic cancers. Hartmann's procedure (for sigmoid cancer) involves the formation of a stoma. Adjuvant chemotherapy (5-fluorouracil or 5FU and folinic acid) is typically reserved for Dukes' C and D. Radiotherapy (preoperative and/or postoperative) may be used to prevent local recurrence.

Name 2 complications of a stoma   ***2 marks***

1. Psychosocial problems, eg body image problems, relationship problems, decreased ability to work, restriction on social activities.

2. Physical problems, eg stenosis of the stoma, prolapse (protrusion) of the stoma, obstruction, parastomal hernia, dehydration and electrolyte disturbance (especially if high output), skin problems (eg infection, ulceration, physical damage caused by frequent removal).

A stoma is a surgically created opening, eg of the bowel, to the body surface, eg colostomy (opens out into the left iliac fossa) and ileostomy (opens out into the right iliac fossa).

What member of the community care team should be involved in Rachel's care? **2 marks**

1. **Stoma care nurse.**

🛈 The stoma care nurse is expert at helping patients to manage their stomas (eg good skin care, fitting secure odourless bags) and advising patients on the physical and pyschosocial problems associated with stomas.

Total: **20 marks**

Further reading

NICE guidelines. *Improving Guidelines in Colorectal Cancers*: www.nice.org.uk

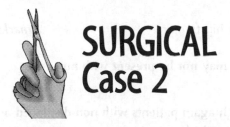

SURGICAL
Case 2

Ethel, a rather frail 86-year-old who resides at Riverside nursing home, is brought into the emergency department after her carers say that she is 'off her legs' since falling out of bed that morning.

List 6 <u>systemic</u> causes of 'off the legs' in elderly people　　　　***3 marks***

'Off the legs' is a common, non-specific presentation in elderly people and may be the result of local (eg osteoarthritis [OA], hip fracture), systemic or psychiatric (eg depression) causes:

1. **Infection, eg urinary tract infection (UTI), pneumonia.**

2. **Anaemia.**

3. **Myocardial infarction (MI).**

4. **Renal failure.**

5. **Electrolyte disturbance, eg hypokalaemia.**

6. **Cerebrovascular accident (CVA).**

7. **Parkinson's disease.**

8. **Cord compression/cauda equina.**

9. **Drugs, eg alcohol, sedatives.**

Your findings on examination of her left leg are consistent with a hip fracture.

QUESTIONS
PAGES 7–10

What findings would be consistent with a hip fracture?   *2 marks*

1. **Leg shortened and externally rotated: may not be present with non-displaced or incomplete fractures**

2. **Patient unable to weight bear, although again patients with non-displaced or incomplete fractures may be able to weight bear.**

3. **Bruising: may not be present with intracapsular fractures because bleeding confined to within the capsule.**

4. **Swelling in the hip region.**

5. **Tenderness over the hip joint (felt in the groin) and greater trochanter.**

6. **Pain on movement of the affected leg.**

7. **Crepitus on movement of the affected leg**

Hip fractures refer to fractures of the proximal femur (see below for classifications). In the UK over 60 000 hip fractures occur per year, in patients of mean age 80 years. The main risk factors are female sex, increased risk of falling and osteoporosis.

You request anteroposterior (AP) (shown below) and lateral X-rays to confirm your diagnosis.

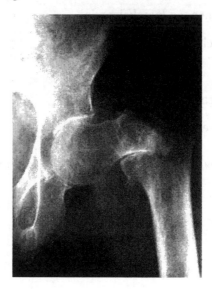

Is this fracture intra- or extracapsular? **2 marks**

1. Extracapsular: displaced intertrochanteric fracture.

Hip fractures are classified as intracapsular or extracapsular, depending on the site of the fracture in relation to the insertion of the capsule of the hip joint (indicated with an arrow) onto the proximal femur. Basal cervical fracture lines tend to be approximately at the level of the insertion of the joint capsule and are classified (and behave) as extracapsular fractures. The classification is important in determining management.

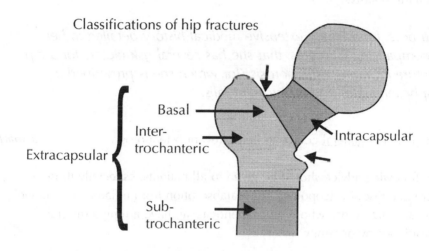

Classifications of hip fractures

Extracapsular { Basal Inter-trochanteric Sub-trochanteric / Intracapsular

Name a late complication of treating intracapsular fractures by internal fixation as opposed to hemiarthroplasty **1 mark**

1. Non-union.

2. Avascular necrosis (AVN) of the femoral head.

The femoral head receives blood from the intramedullary vessels, the trochanteric anastomosis (formed by anastomosis of branches of the gluteal and circumflex-femoral arteries) and the artery of the ligament of the head of femur. Intracapsular fractures may disrupt the former two, such that the blood supply to the head becomes inadequate, causing non-union or AVN (extracapsular fractures are less likely to disrupt the blood supply).

🔹 Intracapsular fractures may be treated by either internal fixation (eg cancellous screws) or hemiarthroplasty of the femoral head. The choice of treatment depends on the patient's age, normal mobility and degree of displacement. Internal fixation is indicated in non-displaced fractures or displaced fractures in younger patients (aim is to try to preserve the head because of the functional deterioration of a hemiarthroplasty and should ideally be done within 6 hours). Hemiarthroplasty is indicated in displaced fractures. If internally fixed, intracapsular fractures are followed up (for 2 years) to exclude AVN or non-union, treatment of which is hemiarthroplasty.

You note, from Ethel's extensive medical history detailed in her accompanying GP notes, that she has several risk factors for a hip fracture including osteoporosis (for which she is prescribed a bisphosphonate) and a history of falls.

Give 3 pieces of <u>general</u> advice to help prevent osteoporosis **3 marks**

🔹 The following advice should be given to <u>all</u> patients, especially those at increased risk of osteoporosis (eg malabsorption from inflammatory bowel disease [IBD], those who are postmenopausal, have a long-term oral steroid therapy or family history):

1. **Increase level of physical exercise.**

2. **Stop smoking.**

3. **Increase dietary calcium intake, eg milk.**

4. **Allow only adequate, safe, sunshine exposure.**

🔹 Osteoporosis is defined as bone density ≥ 2.5 standard deviations (SD) below the bone density of a healthy young adult (osteopenia is bone density -1 to -2.5 SD below normal bone density). The bone that is present is normally mineralised but is deficient in quantity, quality and structural integrity. When it involves the trabecular bone, it increases the risk of crush fractures of the vertebrae; involvement of cortical bone increases the risk of fractures of the long bone. Osteoporosis can be assessed using a DEXA (dual-energy X-ray absorptiometry) scan which quantifies bone density at the proximal femur and spine.

How do bisphosphonates prevent osteoporosis, what is the main side effect and how is this minimised?   **3 marks**

1. **Bisphosphonates inhibit osteoclast activity, thereby preventing bone resorption.**

2. **Oesophageal reactions, eg gastro-oesophageal reflux disease (GORD), dyspepsia, oesophagitis.**

3. **Tablets should be taken while sitting or standing and patients should remain upright for ≥ 1 hour after taking the tablet to prevent oesophageal reflux.**

Bisphosphonates, eg alendronic acid (Fosamax), are indicated in the prophylaxis and treatment of osteoporosis and corticosteroid-induced osteoporosis. They are also used in the treatment of Paget's disease and hypercalcaemia of malignancy.

The orthopaedic surgeon elects to fix Ethel's hip fracture with a dynamic hip screw (DHS) and she is scheduled for surgery the next day.

As the FY1 doctor what 8 things should you ensure before surgery?   **4 marks**

1. **ECG.**

2. **CXR.**

3. **Full blood count (FBC): exclude any anaemia (may require a transfusion before surgery if haemoglobin [Hb] <8 g/dL).**

4. **Urea and electrolytes (U&Es): correct any electrolyte imbalance; exclude impaired renal function.**

5. **Glucose.**

6. **Group and save (or cross-match if Hb <8 g/dL).**

7. **Deep vein thrombosis (DVT) prophylaxis, eg subcutaneous low-molecular-weight (LMW) heparin, aspirin, antiembolic stockings.**

8. **Patient is nil by mouth (NBM), ie on intravenous fluids: *no drip, no hip*.**

9. **Consent.**

10.**Limb is marked: ensures correct hip is operated on.**

🔹 It is the anaesthetist's responsibility to assess the patient's suitability for regional/general anaesthesia partly on the basis of the results of the investigations above.

Surgery is successful and Ethel is encouraged to start partially weight bearing the following day.

Give 4 reasons why Ethel should start weight bearing asap   *2 marks*

1. **Avoids the complications of bed rest, eg DVT, pressure sores.**

2. **Prevents joint stiffness.**

3. **Restores muscle strength.**

4. **Helps regain balance and increases confidence in walking.**

5. **Promotes fracture healing.**

🔹 The management of any fracture involves (a) reduction, (b) fixation and (c) rehabilitation. Weight bearing (which may require a check of the X-ray beforehand) is an important part of the rehabilitation process after a hip fracture. Following internal fixation the patient should sit up in the bed or a chair from postoperative day 1 with partial or full weight bearing on the injured leg asap.

🔹 One in five patients dies within the first year of a hip fracture with one in four elderly patients requiring higher levels of care on discharge.

Total: *20 marks*

Further reading

National Osteoporosis Society. *Primary Care Strategy for Osteoporosis and Falls*: www.nos.org.uk

SIGN. *Prevention and Management of Hip Fracture in Older People*: www.sign.ac.uk/guidelines/fulltext/56

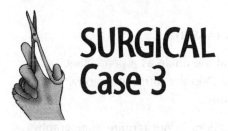

SURGICAL
Case 3

Kristine, a 40-cigarettes-a day publican, is referred by her GP to the peripheral vascular disease (PVD) clinic with a history of muscular cramp-like pain, mainly in one calf, on walking a short distance, which is rapidly relieved by rest.

What is the differential diagnosis for her leg pain?   **2 marks**

When patients present with leg pain on walking that is relieved by rest, the following conditions need to be considered within your differential diagnosis:

1. **Arterial disease, ie PVD.**

2. **Venous disease, eg DVT.**

3. **Musculoskeletal (MSK), eg OA of joints, muscular strain.**

4. **Neuropathic pain, eg cauda equina compression caused by spinal canal stenosis or sciatica.**

5. **Compartment syndrome: swelling of muscles within their rigid osteofascial compartments on exercise as a result of increased perfusion.**

PVD typically causes a cramp-like pain on walking (claudication distance) that is rapidly relieved by rest (intermittent claudication) after which they can walk further. The claudication distance is constant (there are no good days when they can walk further), although if exercise is increased (eg walking up hill) the pain comes on sooner.

On examination, she has absent popliteal and foot pulses in her affected leg.

What non-invasive test confirms the diagnosis of PVD?   **1 mark**

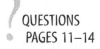

QUESTIONS
PAGES 11–14

1. **Ankle–brachial systolic pressure index (ABSPI).**

🌑 The ABSPI expresses systolic pressure at the ankle as a percentage of the brachial systolic pressure (measured by Doppler ultrasonography): 1 – normal; <0.5 – severe arterial compromise.

🌑 Most patients with intermittent claudication do not require angiography because it is essentially a pre-surgical investigation, although duplex ultrasonography may be used to identify the site of the lesion.

Kristine is discharged back to the care of her GP for treatment of her PVD risk factors.

What are the main <u>modifiable</u> risk factors for PVD?   *2 marks*

1. **Smoking.**

2. **Diabetes mellitus.**

3. **Hypertension.**

4. **Hyperlipidaemia.**

🌑 The management of intermittent claudication involves the modification of PVD risk factors as well as regular exercise and aspirin (see below). Surgical (eg bypass, endarterectomy) or radiological (eg angioplasty ± stenting) intervention is typically reserved for patients with critical ischaemia (see below).

What advice would you give Kristine?   *3 marks*

1. **Stop smoking.**

2. **Take regular aspirin (or clopidogrel if contraindicated).**

3. **Take regular exercise.**

Surgical

- Stopping smoking improves circulation in both the short and the long term (by slowing down the progression of atherosclerosis). The short-term effects of smoking on circulation include increased platelet aggregation, vasoconstriction and hypoxia (resulting from carbon monoxide binding to and reducing the oxygen-carrying capacity of Hb).

- Patients with intermittent claudication have an increased risk of cardiovascular disease and are prescribed aspirin to reduce the risk of cardiovascular events such as MI and CVA.

- Patients should be encouraged to walk to near maximum pain tolerance because this improves symptoms and prevents progression to critical ischaemia by stimulating the development of collateral circulation (although if they get chest pain they should stop immediately).

Twelve months later Kristine is urgently referred back to the PVD clinic describing a history of deteriorating claudication in the same leg, which has recently progressed to nocturnal rest pain. On examination her affected foot shows signs of critical ischaemia.

What are the signs of a critically ischaemic foot?   **4 marks**

1. **Cold.**

2. **Skin discoloration: often purple–blue cyanosed appearance.**

3. **Hair loss.**

4. **Absent foot pulses.**

5. **Prolonged capillary refill time.**

6. **Necrosis/gangrene: usually confined to a toe.**

7. **Ulceration: arterial ulcers typically affect the pressure points of the heel, malleoli and toes, and are described as painful, punched-out lesions.**

8. **Venous guttering: collapsed veins look like pale-blue gutters (veins are normally full).**

9. **Positive Beurger's test: elevation of the leg causes the foot to go white because peripheral arterial pressure can't overcome gravity.**

🔵 Critical ischaemia refers to arterial insufficiency severe enough to threaten the viability of the foot or leg, requiring surgical or radiological intervention (see above).

Why is pain typically worse at night?   *2 marks*

Critical ischaemia is characterised by rest pain which is worse at night as a result of:

1. **Sleep-associated fall in systolic blood pressure.**

2. **Increased warmth of blankets causes peripheral vasodilatation, resulting in a further fall in blood pressure.**

3. **Loss of gravity-dependent circulation.**

🔵 Patients with night pain often relieve their symptoms by sleeping in a chair or with their foot hanging out of the bed.

Kristine undergoes a magnetic resonance angiogram (MRA – shown below) and her occluded artery is treated by percutaneous transluminal angioplasty (PCTA).

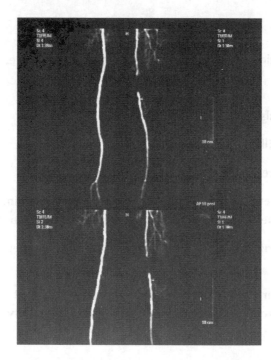

What artery is occluded?   **2 marks**

1. Left (1) superficial femoral artery (1).

ⓘ Angioplasty (± stent) is typically used for stenoses or short occlusions of the iliac or superficial femoral artery. Bypass surgery is reserved for longer occlusions or diffuse disease, using either synthetic or long saphenous venous grafts.

Two years later Kristine presents to the emergency department with features of acute limb ischaemia.

List 6 causes of embolic acute lower limb ischaemia   **3 marks**

1. Atrial fibrillation.

2. MI causing a mural wall thrombus.

3. Subacute bacterial endocarditis (SBE).

4. Aortic or mitral valve disease.

5. Prosthetic heart valves.

6. Patent foramen ovale (paradoxical embolus).

7. Abdominal aortic aneurysm (AAA).

ⓘ Acute ischaemia is caused by either emboli or thrombosis *in situ* (acute-on-chronic ischaemia). It is highly likely that, with Kristine's past history of PVD, her acute limb ischaemia is the result of thrombosis *in situ* rather than an embolic cause.

ⓘ The history (eg recent MI, underlying PVD) and examination (eg heart murmur, state of contralateral pulses) can help identify the underlying cause, which influences treatment: embolectomy or thrombolysis for embolic causes; thrombolysis, angioplasty or bypass surgery for arterial thrombosis.

Give 6 features of acute limb ischaemia   *3 marks*

1. **Pain.**

2. **Pallor.**

3. **Pulseless.**

4. **Perishing cold.**

5. **Paraesthesia: supersedes pain.**

6. **Paralysis: unable to wiggle toes.**

ⓘ Paraesthesia and paralysis are the key to diagnosing <u>complete</u> acute ischaemia, which requires emergency surgical revascularisation within 6 hours in order to salvage the limb (<u>incomplete</u> ischaemia, ie features [1–4], can usually be treated medically in the first instance, eg anticoagulation to prevent propagation of the thrombus and protect the collateral circulation).

Examination is suggestive of complete acute ischaemia. She is given intravenous heparin and taken straight to theatre for revascularisation of her leg.

Name 3 complications of reperfusion   *3 marks*

1. **Reperfusion injury (see below).**

2. **Cardiac arrhythmias: caused by metabolic acidosis and hyperkalaemia.**

3. **Acute renal failure: rhabdomyolysis causes release of myoglobin, which can cause acute tubular necrosis.**

4. **Acute respiratory distress syndrome (ARDS).**

5. **Compartment syndrome: increased capillary permeability and oedema on reperfusion causes muscles to swell within their rigid osteofascial compartments, causing muscle necrosis. Prevented by fasciotomy.**

ⓘ The reintroduction of oxygenated blood after ischaemia causes more damage than ischaemia alone, termed 'reperfusion injury', and is caused by production of highly reactive free radicals.

🔵 Reperfusion washes out the byproducts of anaerobic metabolism (eg lactic acid) and cell lysis (eg potassium, myoglobin), causing arrhythmias, ARDS and acute renal failure.

Total: **25 marks**

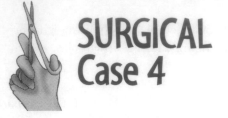

SURGICAL
Case 4

Katie, a 49-year-old art teacher, visits her GP complaining of 'menopausal' symptoms.

What climacteric symptoms may she have?   *2 marks*

1. **Menstrual irregularities.**

2. **Vasomotor symptoms, eg hot flushes, night sweats: caused by disturbance to the hypothalamic thermoregulatory centre.**

3. **Disturbed sleep patterns: may be the result of night sweats.**

4. **Psychological symptoms, eg depression, irritability, lack of concentration, poor memory: these psychological symptoms may result partly from disturbed sleep patterns.**

5. **Vaginal atrophy causing dyspareunia, stress incontinence, UTIs: may respond to topical oestrogens.**

6. **Loss of libido.**

⓵ The climacteric (which spans the age 45–55 years) refers to the period of transition from fertility to infertility and is the result of a decline in circulating oestrogen; this is also responsible for the climacteric symptoms, which may occur before the menopause itself.

⓵ The menopause (commonly misused to describe the climacteric) typically occurs at 51 years (if before 45 years it is termed 'premature'). Any subsequent bleeding is termed 'postmenopausal bleeding', which requires investigation.

She tells you that a friend who is on hormone replacement therapy (HRT) swears by it but is not sure whether it is the best treatment for her.

QUESTIONS
PAGES 15–19

Of what conditions does HRT increase the risk? **2 marks**

1. **DVT/pulmonary embolism (PE) (venous thromboembolism).**

2. **CVA (arterial thromboembolism).**

3. **Cardiovascular disease (CVD) (although increased risk is restricted to first year of use).**

4. **Breast cancer.**

5. **Endometrial cancer.**

6. **Ovarian cancer.**

7. **Alzheimer's disease.**

🜂 The risk of breast cancer is related to the duration of HRT use although this excess risk disappears within about 5 years of stopping. The relative risk of breast cancer using combined HRT is 1.2 after 5 years, increasing to 1.6 after 10 years (women using HRT for > 5 years should be counselled about their increased risks).

🜂 Contraindications to HRT include pregnancy, breast-feeding, CVD, previous DVT/PE, oestrogen-dependent cancers (breast and endometrial), undiagnosed vaginal bleeding (need to exclude endometrial cancer) and active liver disease (affects the pharmacokinetics of HRT).

Which women should receive cyclical progesterone? **1 mark**

1. **Women with an intact uterus.**

🜂 HRT is oestrogen ± progesterone. In women with an intact uterus, addition of cyclical progesterone (for the last 14 days of the cycle causing a withdrawal bleed) reduces the risk of oestrogen-dependent endometrial cancer (although it increases the risk of breast cancer).

It soon becomes obvious that Katie's reluctance for HRT relates to concerns about breast cancer. She wonders why she has not yet been invited for screening.

From what age are women invited to attend the NHS breast screening programme? *1 mark*

1. 50 years.

The NHS breast screening programme was started in 1988. The aim of screening is to detect early, non-palpable, non-invasive disease (70% of screen-detected breast cancers are impalpable), which can be treated by breast conservation. All women aged 50–70 years are invited every 3 years for two-view mammogram of each breast with the option of self-referral for older women (mammography is not considered effective in premenopausal women because of the lower incidence of breast cancer and the increased density of breast tissue).

List 6 criteria used in deciding whether to screen for a disease *3 marks*

1. **Is the disease to be screened an important health problem? Breast cancer affects 1 in 9 women and is a leading cause of cancer death in women.**

2. **Is there a recognisable early stage of the disease? Compared with symptomatic cancers, screen-detected cancers are smaller and more likely to be non-invasive, whereas any invasive cancers are more likely to be better differentiated, of special type and node negative, all of which confer a better prognosis.**

3. **Is there a sensitive and specific (valid) test available for the early detection of the disease? Mammography is 90% sensitive and 95% specific in detecting breast cancer (see below).**

4. **The test must be acceptable, with a high participation rate: 1.5 million women are screened annually (75% of those invited).**

5. **There should be suitable facilities for the diagnosis and treatment of detected abnormalities: any woman with mammographic abnormalities is referred for triple assessment (7% of women are referred at initial screen and 5% on subsequent screening).**

6. **Does screening result in reduced morbidity/mortality?** It is estimated that, since the programme began, screening has resulted in a 10% reduction in the breast cancer death rate (although this is an area of continuing controversy).

7. **There should be appropriate treatment options: see below.**

8. **The benefits of screening must be of an acceptable financial cost:** the annual screening programme costs £52 million (or £35 per woman screened) and detects 10 000 cancers (£5000 per cancer).

🛈 Sensitivity refers to the ability of mammography to detect breast cancer when it is present. Specificity refers to the ability of mammography to identify healthy women as cancer free. Seventy per cent of women referred because of screen-detected abnormalities prove to be clear on further imaging and, of the abnormalities biopsied, 15% are benign.

She then tells you that this morning she found a lump in her left breast and asks you to examine her for breast cancer.

What signs would you look for on breast examination?   *3 marks*

1. **Lump: hard, irregular, fixed, usually painless.**

2. **Breast asymmetry: this can be accentuated by asking her to extend her arms above her head and then placing them on her hips.**

3. **Skin dimpling: tethering of skin to underlying cancer.**

4. **Eczema/ulceration of the areola: Paget's disease (ductal cancer involving the nipple).**

5. **Peau d'orange: oedema of the skin.**

6. **Nipple deviated or inverted.**

7. **Bloody nipple discharge.**

8. **Palpable axillary lymph nodes.**

From the graph below identify which breast lump corresponds to which peak in incidence   *4 marks*

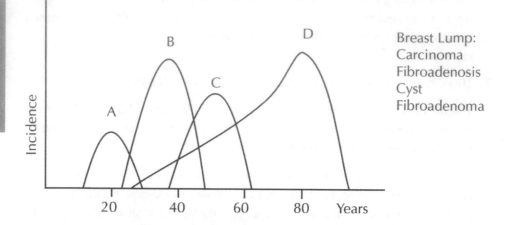

Breast Lump:
Carcinoma
Fibroadenosis
Cyst
Fibroadenoma

Age incidence of common breast lumps

1. **A: Fibroadenoma: most common cause of a breast lump in a young woman.**

2. **B: Fibroadenosis: tender or painful diffuse lumpiness before menstruation.**

3. **C: Cyst.**

4. **D: Carcinoma.**

🛈 Breast cancer (adenocarcinoma arising from the glandular epithelium) is classified as non-invasive (ie ductal and lobular carcinoma *in situ*, not all cases of which progress to invasive cancer) and invasive (penetrates basement membrane of ducts and lobules into surrounding normal tissue). The most common invasive subtype is ductal carcinoma (85%).

On examination you find a lump and, concerned that it may be breast cancer, you urgently refer her for triple assessment.

What are the 3 components of the triple assessment?   *3 marks*

1. **Clinical examination: detects 70% of cancers (as above).**

2. **Imaging (mammogram and/or ultrasound scan [USS]): detects 80% of cancers.**

3. **Cytological assessment (fine-needle aspiration [FNA] or needle core biopsy): detects 95–99% of cancers.**

- On mammography (specialised X-ray image of the breast) fat appears grey whereas denser glandular tissue appears white. Breast cancers have an irregular margin, and are ill defined and dense (whiter than surrounding breast).

- USS involves high-frequency sound waves that enter the breast, some of which are absorbed and some of which reflected back to form an image. Cancers consist of densely packed cells and so block sound wave transmission through the breast; they therefore appear dark (hypoechoic) with a shadow behind them. USS may also be used to guide FNA/core biopsy.

Katie's mammogram and USS are shown, consistent with breast cancer.

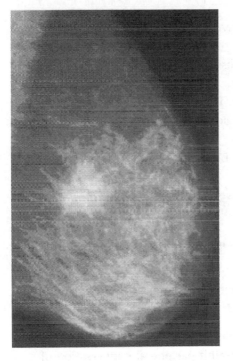 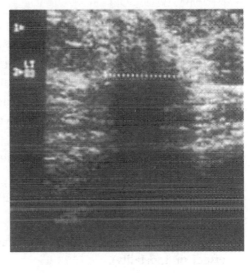

Mammogram (left) demonstrates an irregular mass in the central part of the left breast, which has spicules radiating from it. USS (right) shows a hypoechoic lesion.

Name 4 metastatic sites for breast cancer   *4 marks*

1. **Bone: most common site.**

2. **Lung.**

3. **Liver.**

4. **Brain.**

ⓘ There are two staging classifications for breast cancer: a detailed description by tumour, node status and metastatic parameters (TNM system), which can be amalgamated into four broader stages (UICC system): (I) unfixed, (II) unfixed + positive lymph nodes, (III) fixed (overlying skin or underlying muscle) + positive nodes and (IV) distant metastases.

ⓘ All patients with breast cancer should have an FBC, liver function tests (LFTs), bone profile and CXR. Patients with stage I and II disease have a low incidence of detectable metastatic disease and, in the absence of abnormal symptoms, signs or test results, should not undergo further investigation to assess metastatic disease. Patients with stage III or IV should be considered for bone and liver scans.

List 4 potential treatment options for Katie's breast cancer   *4 marks*

1. **Surgery: wide local excision (breast-conserving surgery [BCS]) or mastectomy.**

2. **Radiotherapy: used after BCS to prevent local recurrence (although has no effect on mortality).**

3. **Cytotoxic chemotherapy, eg CMF (cyclophosphamide, methotrexate, 5FU): used for both adjuvant therapy (before BCS) and metastatic disease.**

4. **Endocrine therapy, eg tamoxifen (oestrogen receptor antagonist) or aromatase inhibitors (eg anastrozole – inhibit peripheral conversation of androgens to oestrogen). Tamoxifen is given to all oestrogen receptor (ER)-positive early breast cancers; aromatase inhibitors are considered first line for ER-positive advanced breast cancers.**

ⓘ Treatment depends on the woman's age and the staging, histological type and biochemical status (eg ER status) of the tumour.

What is a sentinel node? *1 mark*

1. **The sentinel node is the first lymph node that drains an area of tissue (or tumour).**

ⓘ The lymphatic system is a network that returns interstitial fluid back into the systemic circulation. As an area of tissue is drained, the lymphatic fluid flows in an orderly way; the first lymph node through which it flows is termed the 'sentinel node' (and hence breast cancers that metastasise via the axillary lymphatic system will follow a similar course).

What is the advantage of performing a sentinel node biopsy? *2 marks*

1. **It allows axillary nodal status to be assessed without the need for axillary clearance.**

ⓘ Axillary clearance (to both stage the disease and treat the axilla) is considered in all women with invasive breast cancer. However, it is associated with significant morbidity (lymphoedema, shoulder stiffness, reduced range of movement) and, in women with clinically early breast cancer and no palpable nodes, clearance often reveals negative nodes.

ⓘ The sentinel node status is highly predictive of axillary status; only if positive would axillary clearance would be performed. The sentinel node can be identified (and hence sampled) by injection of dye and/or isotope into the peritumoral site, tracing its course into the axilla.

Total: *30 marks*

Further reading

For further information on breast cancer screening you may wish to read the following paper: Blamey R, Wilson A, Patnick J (2000) ABC of breast disease: Screening for breast cancer. *BMJ* 321: 689–93 (freely available at www.bmj.com)

Guidance on the management of the menopause can be found at: www.prodigy.nhs.uk/guidance/menopause

PSYCHIATRIC CASES:
ANSWERS

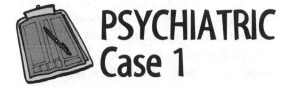

PSYCHIATRIC
Case 1

Lucy visits her GP with symptoms of depression. She has recently separated from her husband and he has moved out of the family home. She tells you she has been feeling down for several months but denies any suicidal thoughts.

Name 8 other symptoms that Lucy may be experiencing　　**4 marks**

1. **Low mood.**

2. **Low self-esteem/self-confidence.**

3. **Feelings of hopelessness and helplessness.**

4. **Pessimism.**

5. **Irritability.**

6. **Guilt.**

7. **Poor concentration.**

8. **Loss of interest/pleasure (anhedonia).**

9. **Fatigue.**

10. **Reduced appetite.**

11. **Reduced weight.**

12. **Reduced libido.**

13. **Insomnia.**

14. **Early morning waking.**

15. **Non-specific physical symptoms, eg headache, back pain.**

ⓘ Symptoms of depression can be classified as either psychological (symptoms 1–9) or physical or somatic (symptoms 10–15).

QUESTIONS
PAGES 23–26

🌀 Depression can be classified as mild (physical symptoms are absent), moderate (physical symptoms are present as are suicidal thoughts) and severe (magnified symptoms of moderate depression with suicidal thoughts prominent ± psychotic symptoms, eg delusions, hallucinations). Typically mild depression is treated in primary care with referral for moderate/severe depression.

Name a class of antidepressant you would consider prescribing in the first instance with 2 examples and 2 associated side effects   *6 marks*

🌀 First-line treatment of depression is either a selective serotonin (5-hydroxytryptamine or 5HT) reuptake inhibitor (SSRI) or a tricyclic antidepressant (TCA). The choice (although in practice SSRIs are usually first choice) depends on patient evaluation, eg suicide risk (SSRIs are less toxic in overdose), concomitant conditions (TCAs should be used with caution in epilepsy and cardiac disease), previous use of antidepressants (use the one that worked last time) and desirability for sedation (use sedative antidepressants if insomnia, eg amitriptyline):

SSRIs:

1. **Examples: citalopram, fluoxetine (Prozac), paroxetine (Seroxat) and sertraline (Lustral).**

2. **Side effects: gastrointestinal (GI) effects (eg nausea and vomiting, constipation and diarrhoea), hypersensitivity reactions (eg rash, urticaria), sexual dysfunction. SSRIs do not have the cardiotoxic or anticholinergic side effects associated with TCAs.**

TCAs:

1. **Examples: lofepramine, amitriptyline, dosulepin (dothiepin), doxepin, imipramine.**

2. **Side effects: anticholinergic side effects (eg drowsiness, dry mouth, blurred vision, constipation, urinary retention), arrhythmias (caused by quinidine-like side action) and seizures.**

Psychiatric

🛈 It takes antidepressants several weeks to work, so the initial therapeutic trial should be at least 4 weeks before changing from TCA to SSRI (or vice versa) or a second drug from the same class. If a patient fails to respond to both TCAs and SSRIs consider psychotherapies, or newer antidepressants, eg mirtazapine. Consider psychiatric referral for patients at risk of suicide, psychotic symptoms, recurrent episodes or refractory depression.

For how long after recovery should the patient continue treatment?   *1 mark*

1. **At least 6 months.**

🛈 Treatment should be continued at least 6 months after symptoms have resolved, after which treatment can be tapered off over 2–4 weeks. This is to prevent relapse in the months after the depressive episode. In patients who relapse, restart treatment with the same antidepressant but continue treatment for longer.

List 2 non-pharmacological treatments of depression   *2 marks*

1. **Cognitive therapy (or cognitive–behavioural therapy or CBT): aim is to correct abnormal ways of thinking so as to improve mood, eg correct false-negative beliefs such as 'nobody likes me'.**

2. **Problem-solving therapy: where the patient and therapist work together to identify key problematic areas and seek to reduce his or her depressive symptoms by resolving these problems.**

3. **Counselling (often provided in a primary care setting).**

4. **Electroconvulsive therapy (ECT): an effective and safe treatment for <u>severe</u> depression.**

🛈 The psychotherapies (1 3), which overlap with each other, are considered effective alternatives or adjuncts to antidepressants in mild and moderate depression.

Several weeks later Lucy presents to the emergency department after taking an overdose of paracetamol. She claims to have taken over 30 tablets (15 g) the night before. A full history, examination and appropriate investigations are taken.

What is considered a potentially fatal dose in adults?   *2 marks*

1. **12 g or 150 mg/kg body weight, whichever is smaller.**

🛈 However, in patients on enzyme-inducing drugs or who are glutathione deplete (see below), death may occur at lower doses (> 75 mg/kg body weight).

Outline 10 questions in the history used to assess suicide risk   *5 marks*

1. **Was the suicide attempt planned or spontaneous?**

2. **Did the patient want to die?**

3. **Was the method used considered potentially lethal by the patient (see above)?**

4. **Did the patient leave a suicide note?**

5. **Did the patient put his or her affairs into order, eg write a will?**

6. **Did the patient take precautions to avoid discovery?**

7. **What was the reason behind the attempted suicide?**

8. **How does the patient feel now, eg still wants to die or feels regret?**

9. **How does the patient feel about the future, eg positive, hopelessness?**

10.**Any previous suicide attempts?**

11.**Any underlying mental illness, eg depression, schizophrenia?**

12.**Any co-morbidities, eg cancer?**

13.**Is the patient currently misusing alcohol or drugs?**

14.**Is the patient socially isolated, eg living alone?**

🛈 Risk factors for suicide include: male, age, substance misuse, underlying physical or mental health problems, social isolation, previous suicide attempts, expressed wish to die.

🛈 Patients treated for attempted suicide should be assessed as to whether they are at risk of future suicide and if so referred to the mental health crisis team (MHCT) or liaison psychiatry service before discharge.

Lucy's 11-hour plasma paracetamol concentration is 160 mg/L which is above the normal treatment line shown on the graph below.

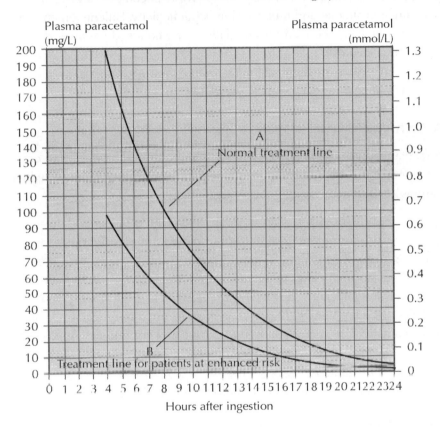

Paracetamol Overdose – Treatment graph

List 2 factors that would put Lucy at enhanced risk **2 marks**

1. **Enzyme-inducing drugs, eg carbamazepine, phenobarbital, phenytoin, rifampicin, alcohol.**

2. **Glutathione deplete, eg people with alcohol problems, anorexia or AIDs.**

Psychiatric

ⓘ Normally paracetamol (acetaminophen) is inactivated by direct hepatic sulfation or glucuronidation. A limited amount undergoes oxidation to form the highly reactive metabolite N-acetylbenzoquineimine, which is subsequently deactivated by glutathione conjugation. If large amounts of paracetamol are ingested the oxidative pathway becomes more significant, depleting glutathione and thus causing hepatotoxicity. Patients on enzyme-inducing drugs (which increases oxidation) or who are glutathione deplete are at enhanced risk.

What is the antidote for paracetamol overdose?   *1 mark*

1. *N*-Acetylcysteine or methionine.

ⓘ Paracetamol overdose antidote is either intravenous N-acetylcysteine or oral methionine, both of which act to replenish hepatic glutathione (which cannot be used because it is not bioavailable).

ⓘ N-Acetylcysteine is given as an infusion. Initially 300 mg/kg body weight is infused in 5% dextrose over a 20-hour period. If the patient presents within 8 hours of overdose, N-acetylcysteine can be delayed until the plasma paracetamol concentration is known because the risk of liver damage is insignificant. Conversely, if presentation is > 8 hours give N-acetylcysteine if a significant dose has been ingested and stop if paracetamol concentrations subsequently indicate no risk. N-Acetylcysteine is an effective antidote up to 24 hours after an overdose (although it is still administered if they present > 24 hours after an overdose and the international normalised ratio [INR] is raised).

Lucy's blood results at the end of the initial antidote treatment are shown below.

Hb	14.1 g/dL	Na+	141 mmol/L	pH	7.37	Bilirubin	16 μmol/L
WCC	8.2 x 10⁹/L	K+	3.9 mmol/L	HCO_3^-	22 mmol/L	ALT	32 IU/L
Platelets	320 x 10⁹/L	Creatinine	91 μmol/L	P_O	11.4 kPa	ALT	29 IU/L
MCV	85 fL	Urea	4.2 mmol/L	P_{CO_2}	4.9 kPa	ALP	134 IU/L
INR	1.7	Glucose	6.4 mmol/L	BE	-1 mmol/L		

ALP, alkaline phosphatase; ALT, alanine transaminase; BE base excess; Hb, haemoglobin; INR, international normalised ratio; MCV, mean cell volume; WCC, white cell count.

Is she <u>medically</u> fit for discharge? Justify your answer **2 marks**

1. **No.**

2. **Her INR is raised. INR is a very sensitive marker of hepatic synthetic function and hence hepatotoxicity; LFTs are less sensitive markers of hepatotoxicity.**

- Before, during and on completion of the course of N-acetylcysteine, FBC (anaemia resulting from haemorrhage), glucose (hypoglycaemia), INR and LFTs, U&Es (renal failure) and arterial blood gases (ABGs) (metabolic acidosis) need to be monitored. If they are normal the patient is medically fit for discharge (although may require an MHCT review). If abnormal continue giving N-acetylcysteine at a rate of 150 mg/kg body weight over 24 hours. If INR <1.4 at 48 hours the patient is medically fit for discharge.

- Criteria for specialist referral: INR > 2 at 48 hours or > 3.5 at 72 hours; creatinine > 200 µmol/L, HCO_3^- <18 mmol/L or blood pH <7.3 at 24 hours.

Total: **25 marks**

Further reading

NICE guideline. *Depression: Management of depression in primary and secondary care*: www.nice.org.uk

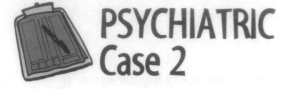

PSYCHIATRIC
Case 2

Sarah is a 21-year-old college student still living at home. Her mother calls out the GP, concerned that Sarah seems to have become very withdrawn, hardly ever leaving her room and refusing to let her in. She has also started wearing a hat made of kitchen foil 'to stop them from hearing what I'm thinking'.

What is a hallucination?   *2 marks*

1. **A sensory experience (or perception experienced as real), in the absence of a stimulus.**

ⓘ The hallucination may be in any modality but in schizophrenia is most commonly auditory (if visual suggests an organic cause). Auditory hallucinations can be in the second person when they take the form of commands to the person. They can also be in the third person when they can be perceived as people either talking about the individual or carrying out a running commentary on his or her actions.

What psychotic symptom is Sarah suffering from?   *1 mark*

1. **Thought broadcasting: she feels that her thoughts are being broadcast out to other people.**

ⓘ Schizophrenia is characterised by delusions, hallucinations and thought disorder (ie psychotic symptoms). Thought broadcasting is an example of a thought disorder; others include thought insertion and withdrawal.

ⓘ Delusions are defined as 'a false unshakeable belief out of keeping with somebody's social, cultural or religious background'. Examples include grandiose, religious and persecutory delusions.

The GP, concerned that Sarah's health is at risk, tries to persuade her to come into hospital for further assessment.

QUESTIONS
PAGES 27–29

What Act may be used to compulsorily treat psychiatric patients?   *2 marks*

1. The 1983 (1) Mental Health Act (1).

🛈 The 1983 Mental Health Act (which applies in England and Wales; Scotland and Northern Ireland have their own Mental Health Acts) is used to carry out both assessment and treatment of patients with psychiatric disorders <u>only</u>; it can't be used to enforce medical treatments even if the patient is detained under the act because of their psychiatric disorder. To use the Mental Health Act requires two medical recommendations from doctors, one of whom is approved under the Mental Health Act and preferably one who is familiar with the patient (eg GP). An application has to be made by an approved psychiatric social worker (ASW).

How long can patients be detained under Section 2 of this Act?   *1 mark*

1. 28 days.

🛈 Section 2 is typically used for the initial assessment when the diagnosis is not clear, or neither doctor has prior knowledge of the patient. Other relevant Sections include: Section 3, which is a treatment order allowing patients to be detained for up to 6 months; Section 4 which is rarely used, but can be applied in an emergency when only one doctor's recommendation is available (typically it is usually converted to a Section 2 order); and Section 5(2) which enables a patient already in hospital as an inpatient to be detained for 72 hours if there would be a risk to the patient him- or herself or to others if he or she were allowed to leave.

Sarah is admitted to the psychiatric hospital where she is subsequently diagnosed with schizophrenia.

What is the differential diagnosis?   *3 marks*

1. Severe depression (depressive psychosis).

2. Bipolar disorder (manic phase).

3. Organic psychosis, eg central nervous system (CNS) tumour or trauma, delirium, dementia, epilepsy, hypothyroidism, systemic lupus erythematosus (SLE).

135

4. Puerperal psychosis.

5. Drug-induced psychosis, either caused by recreational drugs (eg amphetamines) or as a side effect of therapeutic drugs (eg L-dopa, steroids).

🛈 Psychotic symptoms can occur in a wide variety of disorders. Schizophrenia is a clinical diagnosis; some symptoms are more characteristic of schizophrenia than others and a common list of diagnostic symptoms are called first-rank symptoms (although they may occur in other psychotic disorders).

List 4 first-rank symptoms of schizophrenia   *4 marks*

1. Third-person auditory hallucinations, eg voices talking about the person, running commentary.

2. Thought echo, ie voices that echo patient's thoughts.

3. Thought insertion/withdrawal: someone else is inserting or withdrawing thoughts from the patient's head.

4. Thought broadcasting.

5. Passivity of thought, action or feelings, eg patient believes that bodily sensations are controlled by others (somatic passivity).

6. Delusional perception: delusional interpretation of a normally occurring stimulus.

🛈 Schizophrenic symptoms can be broadly divided into positive and negative symptoms. The positive symptoms include hallucinations, delusions and thought disorder; negative symptoms include poor self-care, apathy, social isolation, poverty of speech (little spontaneous speech) and flattening of affect (flattened mood).

🛈 The initial presentation of schizophrenia is usually marked by positive symptoms. With subsequent relapses negative symptoms become more prominent. Some illnesses have an insidious onset with predominantly negative symptoms and it may be difficult to differentiate this from a depressive disorder.

Sarah's psychiatrist prescribes an antipsychotic.

What is the mechanism of action of <u>typical</u> antipsychotics?   *1 mark*

1. Dopamine (D$_2$) receptor antagonist.

🛈 Antipsychotics can be classified as a typical antipsychotic (TAP), eg chlorpromazine or haloperidol, or an atypical antipsychotic (AAP), eg risperidone or clozapine. AAPs have a number of mechanisms of action, eg 5HT receptor antagonists.

🛈 NICE recommend that:

• all newly diagnosed patients with schizophrenia start on an AAP (except clozapine)

• use of an AAP in any acute psychotic episode

• changing from a TAP to an AAP in established schizophrenia is not necessary if symptoms are controlled and side effects acceptable.

List 4 extrapyramidal symptoms (EPSs) of antipsychotics   *4 marks*

Antipsychotics may cause EPSs as a result of dopamine blockade in the extrapyramidal system (less of a problem with an AAP):

1. Parkinsonian symptoms, eg tremor, rigidity, bradykinesia.

2. Acute dystonic reactions: increased muscle tone primarily affecting the face, neck (torticollis), tongue and eyes (oculogyric crises).

3. Akathisia: motor restlessness manifested by the patient either constantly having to move or experiencing a sense of inner restlessness, usually affecting the legs (akathisia may be misdiagnosed as psychotic behaviour).

4. Tardive dyskinesia: most usually a late developing side effect involving involuntary movements of face, tongue, torso or limbs.

🛈 Other complications of antipyschotics include neuroleptic malignant syndrome, which is a rare but life-threatening condition that can occur with any antipsychotic, typically when starting treatment or increasing the dose. Clinical features include fever, muscular rigidity, confusion and autonomic dysfunction (sweating, hypertension, tachycardia).

What type of drug is used to treat EPSs?   *1 mark*

1. Anticholinergics, eg procyclidine.

🛈 EPSs are caused by increased cholinergic activity in the extrapyramidal system resulting from loss of dopaminergic inhibition. With acute dystonia they are administered intramuscularly; otherwise they are given orally. However, anticholinergics are ineffective against tardive dyskinesia (which may be irreversible in up to 50% of affected patients).

Sarah's symptoms are unresponsive to several antipsychotics so eventually she is started on clozapine.

What weekly test will Sarah need?   *1 mark*

1. FBC.

🛈 Clozapine is a very effective AAP (and may improve the negative symptoms). However, it is very expensive and requires daily administration (there is no depot and so compliance becomes an issue) and weekly FBC because it may (rarely) cause agranulocytosis (reduced granular leukocytes, ie basophils, eosinophils, neutrophils).

🛈 NICE recommend that clozapine be reserved for patients unresponsive to two or more antipsychotics.

Total: *20 marks*

Further reading

NICE guidelines. *Schizophrenia: Core interventions in the treatment and management of schizophrenia in primary and secondary care*: www.nice.org.uk

HAEMATOLOGY CASES:
ANSWERS

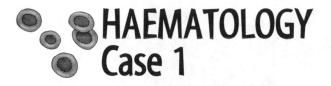

HAEMATOLOGY
Case 1

After a routine blood test that reported lymphocytosis, Andrew, a 54-year-old advertising executive, is recalled by his GP. On examination the only finding of note is cervical lymphadenopathy; he is otherwise asymptomatic.

List 4 causes of lymphadenopathy   **4 marks**

Causes can be classified as either reactive (infective and non-infective) or infiltrative (benign or malignant):

1. **Infective: acute (eg Epstein–Barr virus [EBV], cytomegalovirus [CMV], acute childhood exanthema), chronic (eg tuberculosis [TB], HIV, syphilis).**

2. **Non-infective: sarcoidosis, rheumatoid arthritis (RA), eczema, psoriasis, drug reactions (eg phenytoin).**

3. **Benign, eg lipoidoses (lipid infiltrate).**

4. **Malignant: primary (Hodgkin's disease, non-Hodgkin's lymphoma [NHL], chronic lymphocytic leukaemia [CLL], acute lymphoblastic leukaemia [ALL]), metastatic (eg lung, breast, stomach).**

🕐 Chronic lymphocytic leukaemia is caused by a clonal proliferation of mature B lymphocytes that are functionally defective. It is often diagnosed on a routine FBC (lymphocytes > 5 x 10⁹/L) but may also present with painless lymphadenopathy, anaemia (see below), thrombocytopenia and recurrent infections (caused by neutropenia and reduced immunoglobulin [Ig] levels).

Andrew is referred to the haematology outpatient clinic where he is diagnosed with CLL. As a result of the early stage of his disease he is simply monitored; within 24 months he is symptomatic, has moderate splenomegaly and is anaemic.

? QUESTIONS
   PAGES 33–36   **141**

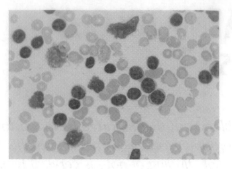

Andrew's peripheral blood film showing stained lymphocytes with thin rims of cytoplasm, coarse condensed nuclear chromatin and the characteristic smear (or smudge) cells.

Name 4 causes of splenomegaly **4 marks**

1. **Infection: acute (eg EBV, SBE), chronic (eg HIV, TB, malaria).**

2. **Inflammation, eg RA (Felty's syndrome), sarcoidosis, SLE.**

3. **Portal hypertension, eg liver cirrhosis.**

4. **Haematological, eg haemolytic anaemia, leukaemia, lymphoma, myeloproliferative disorders.**

ⓘ Splenomegaly typically occurs in the later stages of CLL and is used in clinical staging (based on lymphadenopathy, organomegaly and cytopenia), which helps to determine when to initiate treatment (unnecessary in the early stages of the disease) and in assessing prognosis.

Give 4 reasons why CLL patients may be anaemic **4 marks**

1. **Bone marrow infiltration: may also cause thrombocytopenia and neutropenia.**

2. **Autoimmune haemolysis: CLL is associated with autoimmune cytopenias. Such patients are Coombs' test positive (antibody-coated red blood cells [RBCs]).**

3. **Hypersplenism: as a result of sequestration and destruction of RBCs in enlarged spleen.**

4. **Bone marrow suppression caused by chemotherapy (see below).**

Haematology

Supportive treatment in CLL includes RBC and platelet transfusions, haematopoietic growth factors (eg granulocyte colony-stimulating factor [G-CSF], erythropoietin), infection prophylaxis, eg antibiotics, intravenous immunoglobulin (IVIG), radiotherapy for bulky lymph nodes and splenectomy (eg for massive splenomegaly, autoimmune cytopenias).

As a result of the progressive nature of his disease Andrew's haematologist starts him on cytotoxic chemotherapy with fludarabine.

Name 6 side effects of cytotoxic chemotherapy   *3 marks*

Cytotoxic chemotherapy exerts its effect by inhibiting processes involved in cell division; thus both normal and malignant cells are susceptible to chemotherapy (although malignant cells are more sensitive as a result of increased proliferation or defective DNA-repair mechanisms). Dividing cells in the bone marrow, GI tract, hair follicles and gonads are very sensitive to chemotherapy, causing common side effects (other side effects are drug specific):

1. **Bone marrow suppression causing anaemia, thrombocytopenia (intramuscular injections are contraindicated) and leukopenia (may require prophylactic antibiotics, G-CSF).**

2. **GI symptoms, eg nausea and vomiting, diarrhoea, weight loss, mucositis (oral ulceration).**

3. **Hair loss.**

4. **Hyperuricaemia (see below).**

5. **Infertility: both spermatogenesis and oogenesis are susceptible to chemotherapy.**

6. **Secondary malignancies: caused by DNA damage.**

Chemotherapy may be given orally, parenterally (eg Hickman line) or intrathecally. Most chemotherapy is given in cycles to allow recovery of major organs. Often combination chemotherapy is given to overcome chemoresistance, improve remission rates and increase the cytotoxic effect, eg CVP regimen for CLL combines cyclophosphamide, vincristine (Oncovin) and prednisolone.

What drug is used to prevent tumour lysis syndrome?   *1 mark*

1. **Allopurinol: xanthine oxidase inhibitor (enzyme responsible for conversion of xanthine to uric acid).**

2. **Rasburicase: a newly licensed recombinant urate oxidase which increases uric acid degradation.**

ⓘ Rapid cell death on starting chemotherapy for rapidly proliferating cancers, eg haematological malignancies, can result in hyperuricaemia (and hyperkalaemia), causing renal failure (tumour lysis syndrome). This is prevented by giving allopurinol (or rasburicase) before and during chemotherapy.

After chemotherapy Andrew goes into complete remission (CR). He is entered into the MRC CLL5 trial comparing 'autologous stem cell transfer (SCT) against no treatment following first-line chemotherapy'.

List 6 points you need to inform patients of when entering them into a clinical trial   *6 marks*

1. **Purpose of the trial.**

2. **Probability of allocation to treatment or placebo (or standard treatment).**

3. **What the trial involves.**

4. **Anticipated side effects.**

5. **Risks involved including rare serious risks.**

6. **Ability to withdraw at any time during the trial (for any reason).**

7. **Available expenses (although patients must participate voluntarily without financial inducement).**

8. **Access to notes by third parties (in order to analyse the results of the trial).**

9. **Confirmation that an ethics committee has approved the trial.**

ⓘ First-line treatment of CLL involves either chlorambucil or fludarabine. Second-line therapies include CVP, monoclonal antibodies, eg Campath® (anti-CD52) and rituximab (anti-CD20), and allogeneic SCT.

Against which opportunistic infection are SCT patients given prophylactic co-trimoxazole (Septrin)?   *1 mark*

1. *Pneumocystis carinii* **pneumonia.**

ⓘ *Pneumocystis carinii* may cause pneumonia in patients with suppressed cell mediated immunity (eg SCT, chemotherapy) and is prevented by prophylactic co-trimoxazole (combined sulphonamide and trimethoprim) or nebulised pentamidine.

ⓘ In the early post-SCT period infections are frequent and are prevented by prophylactic antibiotics (eg against staphylococci, *Pseudomonas* sp.), antifungals (eg against *Candida* and *Aspergillus* spp.) and antivirals (eg against herpes simplex virus [HSV] and CMV). CMV is potentially fatal and is regularly screened for using the polymerase chain reaction (PCR).

Give 1 advantage and 1 disadvantage of autologous (self) over allogeneic (donor) SCT   *2 marks*

Advantages:

1. **No risk of introducing latent viral infection from donor into immunocompromised recipient where the virus may become reactivated.**

2. **No risk of graft-versus-host disease (GVHD): caused by donor T cells targeting recipient tissue (where necessary the risk is reduced by post-transplantation immunosuppression with cyclosporin).**

3. **Reduced risk of graft rejection: caused by immunocompetent host cells destroying donor stem cells (also after inadequate stem cell dose and viral infection).**

Haematology

Disadvantages:

1. **No graft-versus-leukaemic effect: donor stem cells eliminate the patient's leukaemia through immunological mechanisms (increases the risk of relapse).**

2. **Risk of contamination of autologous stem-cell product with tumour cells: this is prevented by purging the stem-cell product of tumour cells by negative selection with monoclonal antibodies.**

Autologous SCT involves transplantation with stem cells harvested from the patient's own bone marrow or peripheral blood (PBSCT – the preferred option). It involves four stages:

1. **Harvesting: circulating stem cells are increased by chemotherapy and G-CSF before being harvested from the blood by apheresis.**

2. **Conditioning: high-dose chemotherapy with or without total body radiation is used to ablate the bone marrow.**

3. **SCT: simply involves infusion of stem cells, which relocate to the now empty marrow.**

4. **Post-transplant engraftment: this refers to the production of RBCs, white blood cells (WBCs) and platelets. Typically it takes 1–3 weeks, during which time the patient is supported by RBC and platelet transfusions, infection prophylaxis and G-CSF.**

Total: *25 marks*

Further reading

British Society of Haematology. *Guidelines on the Diagnosis and Management of Chronic Lymphocytic Leukaemia*, available at: www.b-s-h.org.uk

Details on clinical trials for leukaemia including the MRC CLL5 can be found at: www.ctsu.ox.ac.uk

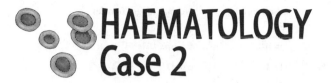

HAEMATOLOGY
Case 2

Lisa, a 22-year-old charity administrator, visits her GP with a 9-month history of progressive fatigue that has become more marked recently. On examination she is clinically anaemic.

Of what other anaemic symptoms may she be complaining?   ***2 marks***

Anaemia may be asymptomatic (especially if chronic) or present with:

1. **Fatigue.**

2. **Shortness of breath.**

3. **Angina.**

4. **Palpitations.**

5. **Faintness.**

6. **Symptoms of the underlying cause, eg RA, peptic ulcer disease.**

7. **Muscle cramps**

🔵 Signs can be divided into general and specific. General signs include pallor, pale conjunctiva, pale palmer creases, tachycardia, systolic flow murmur. Specific signs are associated with the underlying cause, eg koilonychia (iron-deficiency anaemia), glossitis (vitamin B_{12}/folate deficiency), jaundice (haemolysis).

🔵 Causes of anaemia can be broadly classified as (a) reduced production (eg iron deficiency), (b) increased loss (eg GI bleeds) and (c) haemolysis (eg autoimmune).

The GP requests an FBC, reticulocyte count, iron studies, vitamin B_{12} and folate levels, and a peripheral blood film.

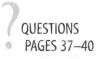

QUESTIONS
PAGES 37–40

147

FBC	Lisa's results	Normal range (female)
Hb (g/dL)	8.8	11.5–16
MCV (fL)	73	76–96
PCV (haematocrit) (%)	27.4	37–47
MCH (pg)	23.3	27–32
MCHC (g/dL)	31.9	30–36
WCC (x10^9/L)	5.2	4–11
Platelets (x10^9/L)	243	150–400

FBC, full blood count; Hb, haemoglobin; MCH, mean cell Hb; MCHC, mean cell Hb content; PCV, packed cell volume; WCC, white cell count.

Name 3 causes of microcytic (low mean cell volume [MCV]) anaemia   **3 marks**

1. **Iron-deficiency anaemia.**

2. **Anaemia of chronic disease (may also cause a normocytic anaemia).**

3. **Thalassaemia.**

4. **Sideroblastic anaemia.**

🛈 Anaemia of chronic disease (which may also cause a normocytic anaemia) is associated with underlying chronic inflammatory diseases and malignancies. It is caused by a reduced RBC lifespan, sequestration of iron by the reticuloendothelial system (RES) and an inadequate erythropoietin (EPO) response to anaemia.

Name 3 causes of macrocytic (high MCV) anaemia   ***3 marks***

1. **Alcohol: most common cause of macrocytosis (ie raised MCV).**

2. **Liver disease.**

3. **Vitamin B$_{12}$ deficiency.**

4. **Folate deficiency.**

5. **Drugs: cytotoxic drugs (eg hydroxyurea), methotrexate (antifolate drug).**

6. **Myelodysplasia.**

7. **Reticulocytosis**

🔵 Macrocytic anaemia can be further divided into megaloblastic (delayed nuclear maturation resulting from defective DNA synthesis, eg vitamin B_{12} or folate deficiency) or non-megaloblastic types, depending on bone marrow findings.

In iron-deficiency anaemia and anaemia of chronic disease indicate ($\uparrow \leftrightarrow \downarrow$) at ? the expected changes   *3 marks*

	Iron-deficiency anaemia	Anaemia of chronic disease	Normal range (females)
Serum ferritin (μg/L)	$\downarrow$	$\uparrow \leftrightarrow$	14–150
Serum iron (μmol/L)	$\downarrow$	$\downarrow$	10–30
TIBC (μmol/L)	$\uparrow$	$\downarrow$	40–75

TIBC, total iron-binding capacity.

🔵 In iron-deficiency anaemia serum iron and serum ferritin (marker of tissue iron stores) levels decrease and total iron-binding capacity (TIBC) increases. With microcytic anaemia and a good history of menorrhagia, you can give oral iron without further investigation – otherwise consider a GI work-up. In anaemia of chronic disease, serum iron and TIBC decrease whereas ferritin may increase (its an inflammatory marker). It responds to treatment of the underlying condition; it doesn't respond to iron supplementation.

Lisa's iron studies indicate that she is iron deficient. She denies menorrhagia and claims to eat a healthy, balanced diet. Her vitamin B_{12} and folate levels and reticulocyte count are shown below.

	Lisa's results	Normal range (females)
Reticulocyte count (x10⁹/L)	32	25–100
Serum vitamin B_{12} (ng/L)	280	160–925
Serum folate (μg/L)	1.9	2.8 13.5

🔵 The reticulocyte count reflects the marrow response to anaemia. The low reticulocyte count (in relation to the anaemia) suggests a problem with RBC production in the marrow, in Lisa's case as a result of iron and folate deficiency.

Haematology

What test is used to distinguish between vitamin B_{12} deficiency caused by malabsorption and lack of intrinsic factor (IF)?   *1 mark*

1. Schilling test.

🛈 Vitamin B_{12} is absorbed in the terminal ileum and requires the presence of IF released by gastric parietal cells. Causes of vitamin B_{12} deficiency (body stores last 2 years) include dietary deficiency (found in meat, fish, eggs and milk, but not in vegetables), IF deficiency (eg pernicious anaemia, gastrectomy) and malabsorption (eg inflammatory bowel disease).

Briefly describe what this test involves   *1 mark*

1. Compares fraction of oral dose of radiolabelled vitamin B_{12} excreted in the urine with and without administration of oral IF.

🛈 Pernicious anaemia is an autoimmune condition causing gastric mucosa atrophy, resulting in IF deficiency. Antibodies to parietal cells (> 90%) and IF (50%) may be present. It presents insidiously with anaemia. If untreated, vitamin B_{12} deficiency may cause neurological changes, eg peripheral neuropathy progressing to involve the posterior and lateral columns of the spinal cord (subacute combined degeneration of the spinal cord).

On further questioning she admits that she has lost weight and passes frequent loose stools. Suspecting malabsorption as the cause of her iron- and folate-deficiency anaemia, Lisa is subsequently diagnosed with coeliac disease.

List 4 other causes of malabsorption   *4 marks*

1. Lack of pancreatic enzymes, eg chronic pancreatitis, pancreatic cancer, cystic fibrosis.

2. Biliary insufficiency, eg intra- and extrahepatic cholestasis, bile salt loss (eg terminal ileal disease), bacterial overgrowth.

3. Small bowel mucosal disease, eg IBD, infection (eg tropical sprue, giardiasis), radiation enteritis, Whipple's disease.

4. Drugs, eg cholestyramine (bind bile salts), metformin, neomycin, laxatives.

5. **Inadequate mixing and intestinal hurry, eg hyperthyroidism, post-gastrectomy.**

🛈 Coeliac disease is caused by gluten-provoked mucosal damage to the proximal small bowel. In adults it may simply present with folate- and/or iron-deficiency anaemia; it doesn't usually cause clinically important vitamin B_{12} deficiency. It can be screened by serum tissue transglutaminase antibodies (tTGs) and confirmed by jejunal biopsy (ie flattened mucosa, villous atrophy, lymphocyte infiltration).

What other condition is associated with folate deficiency? *1 mark*

1. **Neural tube defects (NTDs), eg spina bifida.**

🛈 All women should be prescribed 0.4 mg/day folic acid preconception and first trimester and 5 mg/day if there was a previous NTD.

🛈 Causes of folate deficiency (body stores last 4 months) include dietary deficiency (found in green vegetables), malabsorption (eg coeliac disease), increased demand (eg pregnancy, malignancy) and antifolate drugs (eg methotrexate, anticonvulsants).

Lisa is placed on a gluten-free diet and given iron and folate supplements for 6 months, during which time her blood counts recover.

List 2 side effects of oral iron about which you should warn Lisa *1 mark*

1. **Black stools.**

2. **Constipation.**

3. **Epigastric discomfort.**

4. **Nausea.**

🛈 In iron-deficiency anaemia give ferrous sulphate 200 mg tds. Hb should rise by 1 g/dL per week with reticulocytosis. Continue until Hb is normal and allow an additional 3 months to replenish stores. Failure to respond is usually caused by poor compliance (as a result of side effects), although continued blood loss, malabsorption or misdiagnosis should also be considered.

Name 2 other long-term complications of coeliac disease   *1 mark*

1. **Osteoporosis: as a result of calcium malabsorption.**

2. **Dermatitis herpetiformis: itchy papular vesicular rash.**

3. **Small bowel lymphoma: presents with symptoms of relapsed disease.**

4. **GI carcinoma: increased risk of oesophageal, small bowel and colon cancer.**

5. **Hyposplenism: immunisation against pneumococci recommended.**

ⓘ The risk of these complications is increased in untreated coeliac disease and it is recommended that lifelong follow-up be maintained, eg for symptoms, dietary compliance, blood tests (FBC to exclude anaemia).

Total: *20 marks*

Further reading

British Society of Gastroenterology. *Guidelines for the Management of Patients with Coeliac Disease:* **www.bsg.org.uk**

ENDOCRINOLOGY CASES: ANSWERS

ENDOCRINOLOGY
Case 1

Andy, a 47-year-old estate agent, visits his GP complaining of general tiredness. He's a non-smoker but admits to eating and drinking to excess. On examination he weighs 95 kg and his height is 1.72 m; BP is 154/92 mmHg.

Calculate his body mass index (BMI) **1 mark**

1. 32, ie [weight (kg)]/[height (m)]²ı95/(1.72)² = 32

🛈 Obesity (ie BMI > 30) is a risk factor for the development of type 2 diabetes. In obese patients with type 2 diabetes, weight loss improves glycaemic control and reduces the risk of diabetic complications. In obese patients who are unable to lose weight by lifestyle changes, consider anti-obesity drugs, eg orlistat (reduces dietary fat absorption) or sibutramine (centrally acting appetite suppressant).

Urine dipstick is ++ for glucose.

How would you confirm the diagnosis of diabetes? **2 marks**

1. **Random plasma glucose ≥ 11.1 mmol/L or**

2. **Fasting plasma glucose ≥ 7.0 mmol/L.**

🛈 If the patient is asymptomatic repeat the test, but if borderline perform an oral glucose tolerance test (OGTT) with 75 g glucose. A 2-hour plasma glucose ≥ 11.1 mmol/L confirms the diagnosis.

List 4 other presenting symptoms of type 2 diabetes **4 marks**

1. **Thirst.**

2. **Polyuria/nocturia.**

? QUESTIONS
PAGES 43–45

3. **Blurred vision: caused by glucose-induced changes in lens refraction.**

4. **Infections, eg candida infection (thrush), boils.**

5. **Weight loss (although conversely may also get weight gain).**

6. **Complications of type 2 diabetes, eg CVA, CVD, neuropathy (foot ulcers).**

7. **Hyperglycaemic, hyperosmolar, non-ketotic (HONK) coma.**

ⓘ HONK affects only patients with type 2 diabetes, causing dehydration as a result of severe hyperglycaemia (typically > 35 mmol/L) without acidosis (absence of ketone bodies). Diabetic ketoacidosis (DKA) affects type 1 diabetes only, although treatment for both will require fluids and insulin.

Initially Andy attempts to manage his diabetes mellitus by diet and exercise alone but this fails to control his hyperglycaemia.

On what hypoglycaemic agent would you start Andy?   *1 mark*

1. **Metformin (a biguanide).**

ⓘ Metformin acts by increasing insulin sensitivity and decreasing hepatic gluconeogenesis. It is the first-line treatment in type 2 diabetes, in particular in obese patients, because it doesn't promote weight gain. In non-obese patients or patients contraindicated/unable to tolerate metformin, use sulphonylureas (eg gliclazide) which increase insulin secretion. Use in combination if single therapy is inadequate.

ⓘ Other add-on hypoglycaemia agents include acarbose, which delays digestion and absorption of starch, and glitazones, which act by decreasing peripheral insulin resistance. Insulin is indicated if optimal oral hypoglycaemia combination therapy is inadequate.

Andy is reviewed 6 monthly to monitor his glycaemic control and assess the development of any diabetic complications.

How do you assess long-term glycaemic control?   *1 mark*

1. **HbA1c.**

🔴 HbA1c (glycated haemoglobin) indicates average glucose concentrations over the last 8 weeks (ie half-life of RBCs). The recommended target is 6.5–7.5% and levels should be measured every 2–6 months depending on glycaemic control.

Andy's fasting lipids are measured: total cholesterol (TC) 6.34 mmol/L, LDL 4.22 mmol/L, HDL 1.26 mmol/L, triglycerides 2.4 mmol/L.

Calculate his 10-year coronary heart disease (CHD) risk   ***2 marks***

1. 15%: non-smoking man with diabetes aged between 45 and 54 years with systolic BP of 154 mmHg and TC:HDL of 5.

🔵 The CHD risk prediction charts are found at the back of the *British National Formulary* (BNF) and are used to estimate the risk of CHD (ie non-fatal MI, coronary death, new-onset angina) in patients with <u>no</u> previous history of CVD. In patients with diabetes mellitus, they are used to help guide treatment of coexisting hypertension (see below) and hyperlipidaemia; in patients with raised cholesterol (TC ≥ 5 mmol/L or LDL ≥ 3 mmol/L) prescribe a statin if rate of 10-year CHD risk is ≥ 15%.

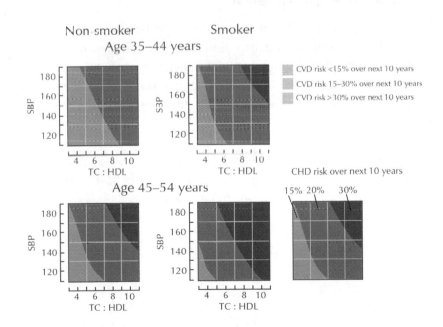

How do you screen for diabetic renal disease? *2 marks*

1. **Urinary albumin:creatinine ratio (ACR) or**

2. **Urinary albumin excretion in 24 hours.**

🔵 The ACR is usually used because it can be done on a 'spot' of urine.

🔵 Microalbuminuria is the earliest indicator of diabetic nephropathy and is defined as ACR ≥ 2.5 mg/mmol (men) or ≥ 3.5 mg/mmol (women) or urinary albumin excretion of 30–300 mg/24 h. Urinary albumin excretion of > 300 mg/24 h indicates macroalbuminuria and should lead to a full assessment of renal function. Treatment of microalbuminuria (which indicates an increased risk of end-stage renal disease and CVD) involves good glycaemic control, treatment of blood pressure (BP) (see below) and angiotensin-converting enzyme (ACE) inhibitor or angiotensin II receptor antagonist (even if normotensive as protects the kidneys).

What is the first-line treatment of hypertension in the presence of diabetic renal disease? *1 mark*

1. **ACE inhibitor or**

2. **Angiotensin II receptor antagonist.**

🔵 Target BP in patients with diabetes mellitus and 10-year rate of CHD risk ≥ 15% depends on whether microalbuminuria is present (≤ 135/75 mmHg) or absent (≤ 140/80 mmHg). For patients with microalbuminuria use ACE inhibitor or angiotensin II receptor antagonist as first-line therapy; for other patients use thiazide, β blocker or ACE inhibitor.

Andy's feet are examined: he has bilateral foot pulses but is unable to perceive the pressure from a 10 g monofilament and so is at increased risk of developing a 'diabetic foot'.

Endocrinology

List 4 pieces of preventive foot care advice   *4 marks*

1. **Wash and inspect feet daily.**

2. **Use creams/lotions to prevent dry skin/callus formation.**

3. **Always have feet measured when buying shoes.**

4. **Avoid walking barefoot.**

5. **Avoid thermal injury, eg from hot water bottles.**

6. **Seek medical attention for any foot injury (however trivial).**

7. **Avoid self-treatment of corns, calluses or other foot problems.**

Diabetic foot problems, eg ulceration, are caused by neuropathy (causing insensitivity with resulting trauma) and/or peripheral vascular disease. Feet should be inspected annually: signs of neuropathy include dry skin and callus formation at pressure areas; inability to perceive a 10 g monofilament is a sensitive indicator of an 'at-risk' foot. Foot pulses should also be assessed. The best treatment is prevention through good foot care, targeting those at increased risk.

As part of his diabetes review, Andy also attends the local optometrist (report as follows): bilateral microaneurysms and microhaemorrhages present, extensive hard exudates noted. No cotton-wool spots detected. No new vessel formation. Visual acuity (while wearing spectacles): 6/6 (left), 6/6 (right).

Classify Andy's diabetic retinopathy   *2 marks*

1. **Background retinopathy.**

Diabetic retinopathy can be classified as:

- Background retinopathy: dots (microaneurysms), blots (microhaemorrhages) and hard exudates. Refer to ophthalmologist if within one disc diameter of macula.

- Pre-proliferative retinopathy: as above but also cotton-wool spots (retinal infarcts). Refer to ophthalmologist.

- Proliferative retinopathy: new vessels form on the retina which may bleed or cause retinal detachment. Urgent referral, eg for laser treatment.

ⓘ All patients with diabetes should be screened annually, eg by an optometrist. Good glycaemic control and treatment of hypertension and hyperlipidaemia delays the onset of retinopathy and can slow its progression.

Total: *20 marks*

Further reading

NICE guidelines 2002. *Management of Type 2 Diabetes*: **www.nice.org.uk**

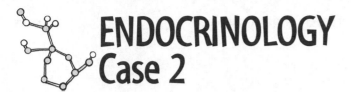

ENDOCRINOLOGY
Case 2

As the surgical FY1 on call you are bleeped to see Zoe, an orthopaedic patient, 2 days after a total hip replacement, with the biochemical results shown below.

	Zoe's results	Normal range
Na$^+$ (mmol/L)	124	135–145
K$^+$ (mmol/L)	4.3	3.5–5
Urea (mmol/L)	3.2	2.5–6.7
Creatinine (µmol/L)	88	70–150
Albumin (g/L)	37	35–50
Glucose (mmol/L)	5.2	4–6

Give 2 common causes of iatrogenic hyponatraemia on the wards   ***2 marks***

1. **Diuretics.**

2. **Inappropriate intravenous fluids, eg excessive intravenous dextrose (dehydration as a result of inadequate fluids tends to cause hypernatraemia).**

Normal postoperative fluid requirement is 2–3 L/24 h which allows for urinary, faecal and insensible losses (although this may need to be increased, eg as a result of losses from surgical drains or operative losses). A standard fluid regimen is 2 L 5% dextrose with 1 L 0.9% saline/24 h (plus 20 mmol/L K$^+$). However, patients at increased risk of hyponatraemia (eg on thiazide diuretics, low Na$^+$ preoperatively and females) may require more saline.

It is worth noting that Na$^+$ may be artefactually low if the blood is taken from an arm with a fluid intravenous drip.

One of the medical students on your ward suggests giving Zoe hypertonic intravenous saline to correct her low Na$^+$.

QUESTIONS
PAGES 46–48

Give 2 clinical features of <u>severe</u> hyponatraemia **2 marks**

1. **Confusion.**

2. **Seizures.**

3. **Coma.**

ℹ️ Hyponatraemia is usually asymptomatic with plasma Na^+ >125 mmol/L; symptoms associated with moderate hyponatraemia (<125 mmol/L) include headaches, lethargy, nausea and muscle weakness. Confusion, seizures and eventually coma are associated with severe hyponatraemia (<115 mmol/L) and are the result of the movement of water into brain cells in response to the fall in extracellular osmolality.

ℹ️ Severe hyponatraemia is prevented by monitoring U&Es pre- and postoperatively (don't ignore low Na^+), avoiding giving dextrose without intravenous saline and retaining a high level of suspicion for odd CNS signs.

Would you give Zoe hypertonic saline? What is the main risk? **2 marks**

1. **No.**

2. **May cause central pontine myelinolysis.**

ℹ️ A rapid rise in extracellular osmolality, in particular in patients with compensated hyponatraemia, will result in severe shrinking of brain cells, causing central pontine myelinolysis (CNS demyelination particularly involving the pons), which is potentially fatal. In <u>severe</u> hyponatraemia (seizures, coma) consider hypertonic (1.8–4.5%) saline (although this should be given slowly, ie <70 mmol Na^+/h) and in aliquots to increase plasma Na^+ to >125 mmol/L (this should be initiated only by your senior). Avoid increasing the Na^+ by more than 12 mmol/L per 24 h.

You assess Zoe to determine whether she is dehydrated or fluid overloaded.

How would you assess Zoe's fluid balance? **4 marks**

Endocrinology

1. **Signs of fluid overload: (JVP (jugular venous pressure), peripheral oedema, pulmonary crepitations (pulmonary oedema).**

2. **Signs of dehydration: ↑HR (heart rate), ↓BP, postural hypotension, ↓skin turgor, dry mucous membranes, raised urea.**

3. **Fluid chart: is the patient receiving appropriate intravenous fluids?**

4. **Urinary output: in catheterised patients this should be charted.**

🔵 When assessing a patient with hyponatraemia the <u>key</u> question is whether they are hypovolaemic, normovolaemic or hypervolaemic because this will help determine the underlying cause and its subsequent treatment (see below).

Name 4 causes of hyponatraemia in fluid-overloaded patients   *2 marks*

1. **Cardiac failure.**

2. **Oliguric renal failure.**

3. **Liver failure.**

4. **Nephrotic syndrome.**

5. **Excessive intravenous dextrose.**

🔵 In hypervolaemic patients, hyponatraemia is simply a result of dilution by the excess total body water (ie dilutional hyponatraemia).

How would you manage hyponatraemia in such patients?   *1 mark*

1. **Fluid restriction.**

🔵 If the patient is clinically hypervolaemic no further investigations are necessary and the hyponatraemia can simply be corrected by fluid restriction (0.5–1.0 L/day). If necessary, acute dilutional hyponatraemia may be treated with 0.9% intravenous saline and furosemide.

How would you exclude renal Na$^+$ loss in dehydrated patients?   *1 mark*

1. **Measure the urinary sodium.**

Endocrinology

🛈 If the patient is dehydrated to determine whether Na^+ is being lost through the kidneys (eg Addison's disease, diuretic excess, osmolar diuresis) or elsewhere (eg diarrhoea and vomiting, burns), measure urinary Na^+; urinary levels > 20 mmol/L indicate that Na^+ (and water) is being lost through the kidneys.

🛈 If dehydrated, correct hyponatraemia by giving 0.9% intravenous saline.

What other electrolyte abnormality would you expect in Addison's disease?   *1 mark*

1. Hyperkalaemia.

2. Raised urea.

🛈 Addison's disease is caused by adrenal insufficiency (glucocorticoid, mineralocorticoid, sex hormone insufficiency). The aldosterone insufficiency causes renal Na^+ loss (and subsequent hypovolaemia); hyperkalaemia is the result of loss of aldosterone-mediated renal K^+ excretion. It is diagnosed by a short Synacthen (ACTH) test, measuring plasma cortisol at baseline and 30 minutes after intravenous Synacthen.

Zoe is neither dehydrated nor fluid overloaded so you request a urinary Na^+ and osmolality, which are reported as 32 mmol/L and 400 mosmol/L, respectively.

Calculate Zoe's plasma osmolality   *2 marks*

1. 265, ie 2(124 + 8.6) + 3.2 + 5.2.

🛈 Normal plasma osmolality is 280–300 msmol/L. It can be calculated from: $(2[Na^+ + K^+]) + [urea] + [glucose])$.

What is the likely cause of her hyponatraemia?   *1 mark*

1. Syndrome of inappropriate antidiuretic hormone secretion (SIADH).

🛈 Surgical stress may cause a transient SIADH postoperatively. SIADH cannot be diagnosed in patients who are hypovolaemic (which stimulates physiological ADH release), hypervolaemia or on diuretics. The diagnosis requires hyponatraemia (typically Na+ <125 mmol/L), low plasma osmolality (typically <270 msmol/L), and concentrated urine (Na+ > 20 mmol/L, urine osmolality > plasma osmolality).

How could you treat her hyponatraemia?   *2 marks*

1. **Fluid restriction.**

2. **Demeclocycline: inhibits actions of ADH (only given if patient doesn't respond to fluid restriction).**

🛈 Fluid restriction is usually sufficient by itself to elevate plasma Na+ to safe levels.

Total: *20 marks*

Endocrinology

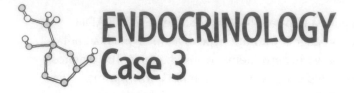

ENDOCRINOLOGY
Case 3

Jack, aged 15, is concerned about his height. He is the shortest in his class and although he enjoys football he finds that he can't keep up with the much bigger boys in his year. His parents, worried about his growth, have taken regular measurements of his height over the past 5 years, as shown below.

Age (years)	Height (cm)	Age (years)	Height (cm)
10	134	13	145
11	138	14	147
12	142	15	149

His parents are of average height: his dad is 172 cm and his mum 164 cm.

Plot Jack's height measurements on the growth chart   ***3 marks***

QUESTIONS
PAGES 49–51

⊕ Short stature is defined as subnormal height related to other children of the same sex and age. Usually the 2nd or 0.4th centile of the growth curve is selected as the cut-off point. During childhood there are two growth spurts: the first, during the infantile years, is largely dependent on good nutrition, emotional nurturing and normal thyroid function; the second occurs during puberty, when sex steroids stimulate an increase in growth hormone secretion from the pituitary. Sex steroids also have a direct effect on bone growth.

Why is it important to know the parents' heights?   ***2 marks***

1. The parents' heights give an indication of Jack's adult height potential.

⊕ Jack's adult height potential can be calculated according to the Adult Height Potential Calculation Table (this is found at the top of growth charts).

a	Father's height	172 cm
b	Mother's height	164 cm
c	Sum of (a) and (b)	336 cm
d	(c) divided by 2	168 cm
e	(d) + 7 cm (MPH)	175 cm
f	MPC – nearest centile	40th centile
g	TCR (MPH ± 10cm)	87th centile–4th centile

MPC, midparental centile; MPH, midparental height; TCR, target centile range.

⊕ This shows that, if he follows his genetic growth pattern, he should reach 175 cm as an adult (his midparental height or MPH). His midparental centile or MPC is the 40th centile and the range between 87th centile and 4th centile indicates his target centile range (TCR). He should be growing within the TCR from the age of 2 years on or parallel to one of the printed centile lines.

Apart from being small, Jack also seems to be a slow developer. A lot of his friends are already shaving and their voices have broken, whereas Jack has no pubertal features yet.

Describe the hormone axis that regulates puberty   *2 marks*

1. **Puberty is triggered by an increase in gonadotrophin-releasing hormone (GnRH) secretion from the hypothalamus.**

ⓘ GnRH stimulates the pituitary gland to release two gonadotrophins: luteinising hormone (LH) and follicle-stimulating hormone (FSH). LH stimulates the testes to produce testosterone and the ovaries to produce oestrogen. FSH stimulates the Sertoli cells to produce sperm and in females it stimulates follicular development.

ⓘ The pituitary gland secretes three other hormones that interact with sex hormones and affect growth: ACTH which stimulates secretion of androgens from the adrenal gland, thyroid-stimulating hormone (TSH) and growth hormone (GH). The increased level of sex hormones and GH triggers two sets of body changes: development of secondary sexual characteristics and a much broader set of changes in brain, muscles, bones and other organs.

What is the first sign of puberty in boys?   *2 marks*

1. **Testicular enlargement (> 4 mL): can be measured by an orchidometer.**

ⓘ The mean age of puberty onset in males is 11.5 years. In females the mean age is 11 years of which the first sign is breast bud enlargement.

What is the name of the puberty staging system?   *1 mark*

1. **Tanner staging system.**

ⓘ Pubertal development can be assessed according to the Tanner stages of puberty. Pubertal changes in breast, pubic hair and genitalia follow a defined sequence of changes, assigned Tanner stages I–V.

What non-invasive investigation can be used to assess growth in Jack?   *1 mark*

1. X-ray of hand and wrist: used to assess skeletal maturation.

🔘 The pattern of maturation of the growth plates (epiphyses) of the radius, ulna, carpals, metacarpals and phalanges is compared with standards derived from healthy children. The appearance of the epiphysis is given a numerical value. A 'bone age' is then calculated from the total of these, which can be compared with the child's chronological (actual) age.

🔘 Children with short stature can have a delay in bone age of several years. This indicates that the child is likely to continue to grow for longer than average and this may enable 'catch-up growth' to occur.

🔘 A non-invasive investigation in girls with short stature is a pelvic USS to assess uterine size, configuration and endometrial thickness.

Which diagnosis is important to exclude In short females with no signs of puberty? **2 marks**

1. Turner syndrome.

🔘 Turner syndrome is a chromosomal disorder resulting from absence or abnormality of the second X chromosome, characterised by short stature and absence of pubertal development and infertility. Diagnosis is conformed by chromosomal analysis (karyotype). Other features associated with Turner syndrome are webbing of the neck, broad chest with widely spaced nipples, wide carrying angle (cubitus valgus), congenital heart defects (especially aortic coarctation), renal abnormalities, shortening of the fourth and fifth metacarpals and metatarsals, and normal intelligence. Short stature in Turner syndrome is caused by a reduced growth rate in childhood and the lack of a pubertal growth spurt as a result of ovarian dysgenesis. Three treatments are used to promote growth – GH, oxandrolone (anabolic steroid) and oestrogen – increasing final height by about 8 cm on average. Apart from stimulating growth, oestrogen is also used to initiate puberty.

What is the most likely cause of Jack's short stature? **2 marks**

1. Constitutional delay of growth and puberty.

ⓘ Constitutional delay of growth and puberty is a common condition in which short stature occurs together with delayed pubertal development in otherwise healthy teenagers. It is often familial and is more common in boys than in girls. It is a variation in the timing of puberty and the child often reaches a normal final height. It can produce extreme anxiety, particularly in boys. Management is reassurance that puberty will soon begin. After the age of 14 years, puberty may be induced using sex steroids.

Give 5 other causes of short stature   *5 marks*

1. **Familial: most children with short stature will have short parents. Check with the Adult Height Potential Calculating Table that the child is growing within his TCR.**

2. **Endocrine disorders, eg GH deficiency (very short stature and markedly delayed bone age), hypothyroidism.**

3. **Chronic disease, eg cardiac disorders, coeliac disease, Crohn's disease, chronic renal failure, anorexia, cystic fibrosis. These children are usually short and underweight.**

4. **Skeletal dysplasias: abnormal bone development should be considered when bone age is not delayed in relation to chronological age, eg in achondroplasia, osteogenesis imperfecta. Also look for characteristic features such as a disproportion between spine and leg length.**

5. **Steroid treatment: corticosteroid therapy is a growth suppressant.**

6. **Chromosomal disorders, eg Turner syndrome, Down syndrome, Noonan syndrome, Russell–Silver syndrome.**

7. **Psychosocial deprivation: these children often show a fast catch-up growth when placed in a better environment.**

8. **Gonadal failure: the testes or ovaries do not respond to the stimulus of gonadotrophins.**

Total: *20 marks*

EMERGENCY MEDICINE CASES: ANSWERS

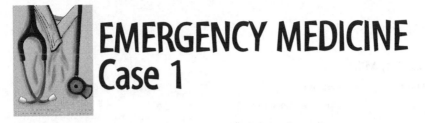

EMERGENCY MEDICINE
Case 1

Gary, a 23-year-old man, is brought into the emergency department after a high-speed road traffic accident (RTA). He has sustained trauma to the left side of his head and has a reduced level of consciousness.

List 3 causes of secondary brain injury   **3 marks**

The aims of managing head injury is to prevent secondary brain injury caused by raised intracranial pressure (ICP):

1. **Blood loss after associated injuries causing ischaemic cerebral oedema.**

2. **Hypoxia and hypercapnia (eg as a result of seizures, chest injury) causing hypoxic and hypercapnic cerebral oedema.**

3. **Infection (eg via skull fracture) causing inflammatory oedema.**

4. **Intracranial haemorrhage causing localised pressure effects and ↑ICP.**

⊕ Secondary brain injury is prevented by managing the patient's ABCs, ie maintaining the airway (although with immobilisation of the neck until a potential cervical spine fracture has been cleared; if the Glasgow Coma Score [GCS] is 8 the patient will require intubation), high-flow O_2 (consider hyperventilating so hypocapnic) and correction of any hypovolaemia. Patients with skull fractures should receive intravenous antibiotics and any seizures should be treated with diazepam. Intracranial haemorrhage may require drainage.

Gary's neck is immobilised, his ABCs are stabilised and an assessment of his neurological status undertaken. His GCS is assessed as follows: his eyes open to pain, he localises pain and his speech is confused.

QUESTIONS
• PAGES 55–57

173

Calculate Gary's GCS   *2 marks*

1. 11/15: E2, V4, M5.

Component	Response	Score
Eye response	Open spontaneously	4
	Open to verbal command	3
	Open to pain	2
	No response	1
Verbal response	Oriented	5
	Confused conversation	4
	Inappropriate speech	3
	Moaning	2
	None	1
Motor response	Obeys command	6
	Localises pain	5
	Withdraws to pain	4
	Abnormal flexion, ie pressure on nail bed causes upper limbs to flex and adduct.	3
	Abnormal extension, ie pressure on nail bed causes upper limbs to extend, adduct and semipronate	2
	No response to pain	1

ⓘ The GCS is a reliable, objective way of recording a patient's conscious state. In a patient with stabilised ABCs a deteriorating GCS is a medical emergency typically caused by ↑ICP. Raised blood pressure and bradycardia (Cushing's response) and fixed, dilated pupils are all signs of ↑ICP. Mannitol is an osmotic diuretic that can help reduce ↑ICP while awaiting further management.

A full examination reveals that Gary has sustained no other major injuries.

List 4 signs on examination of a basal skull fracture   *2 marks*

1. Bilateral orbital bruising, ie panda eyes.

2. Subconjunctival haemorrhage (with no posterior margin evident).

3. **Battle's sign, ie bruising over the mastoid process (this is a late sign).**

4. **Haemotympanum: blood behind the eardrum.**

5. **Otorrhoea, ie cerebrospinal fluid (CSF) discharge from the ears.**

6. **Rhinorrhoea, ie CSF discharge from the nose.**

🌑 Clinical evidence of a skull base fracture is an indication for a skull X-ray (AP, lateral and Towne's views) as are ↓GCS, neurological deficits, scalp wounds and obvious skull fractures (although with serious head injury a CT scan will supersede X-rays).

🌑 Other investigations may include FBC, cross-match, U&Es, glucose, ABGs, clotting screen and radiology (CXR, pelvic X-ray, C-spine X-ray) as indicated.

Other than ↓GCS list 6 other criteria under which you would admit a patient following a head injury   ***3 marks***

1. **History of loss of consciousness.**

2. **History of amnesia (anterograde ± retrograde amnesia).**

3. **History of alcohol ingestion.**

4. **Focal neurological deficit, eg hemiparesis, diplopia.**

5. **Suspected open or depressed skull fracture.**

6. **Penetrating injury.**

7. **Any sign of basal skull fracture.**

8. **Post-traumatic seizure.**

9. **Vomiting.**

10. **Dangerous mechanism of injury, eg thrown from car.**

11. **Coagulopathy, eg current treatment with warfarin.**

12. **Lack of responsible adult in attendance to observe patient on discharge.**

13. **Suspicion of non-accidental injury in children.**

Emergency Medicine

List 6 regular observations that Gary should undergo   **6 marks**

ⓘ Every head-injured patient requires regular neurological observations in order to detect any complications at an early stage:

1. **GCS: see above.**

2. **Pupil size and response to light: fixed, dilated pupil(s) is a false localising sign indicating ↑ICP.**

3. **Limb power: assessment of any focal neurological deficit.**

4. **BP: raised BP may indicate ↑ICP (Cushing's response); reduced BP may indicate hypovolaemia from other injuries.**

5. **Pulse: bradycardia may indicate ↑ICP (Cushing's response) and tachycardia may indicate hypovolaemia from other injuries.**

6. **Respiratory rate: a reduced respiratory rate may reflect CNS depression caused by ↑ICP.**

   Gary's GCS continues to deteriorate so he undergoes an urgent CT scan of his head.

Describe 2 abnormalities seen on his CT scan   **2 marks**

1. **A convex area of high attenuation (or hyperdense area consistent with fresh blood) is seen to extend from the inner layer of the skull on the left.**

2. **This causes a mass effect with midline shift.**

3. **A small area of low attenuation (or hypodense area) is seen peripheral to this.**

ⓘ No skull fracture is evident although air within the skull vault (small area of low attenuation) is in keeping with a skull fracture.

Gary's brain CT scan is shown.

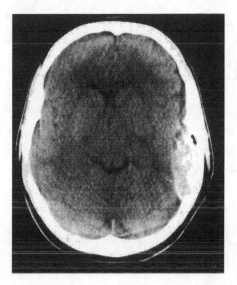

What is the diagnosis? **1 mark**

1. Extradural haemorrhage.

● Classically an extradural haemorrhage appears convex because the dura mater is firmly attached at the suture lines, whereas a subdural haemorrhage appears concave. However, this distinction is not always evident.

● An extradural haemorrhage is caused by tearing of arteries in close proximity to the skull, eg tearing of the anterior branch of the middle meningeal artery may be caused by fracture to the temporal bone.

What further course of action should be undertaken? **1 mark**

1. Urgent neurosurgical referral.

● Intracranial haemorrhage causes localised pressure effects and generalised ↑ICP and may require surgical drainage.

Total: **20 marks**

Further reading

NICE guidelines. *Head Injury: Triage, assessment, investigation and early management of head injury in infants, children and adults*: **www.nice.org.uk**

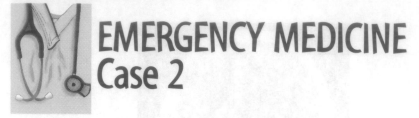

EMERGENCY MEDICINE
Case 2

Rob, a 26-year-old PE teacher, is refereeing a game of football when he complains of a severe occipital headache before vomiting and collapsing on the playing field.

What is the differential diagnosis of a severe headache?   *2 marks*

1. **Subarachnoid haemorrhage (SAH).**

2. **Meningitis.**

3. **Encephalitis.**

4. **Migraine.**

5. **Intracranial venous thrombosis, eg sagittal sinus thrombosis.**

6. **Subdural haematoma.**

7. **Benign thunderclap headache.**

8. **Head injury.**

9. **Temporal arteritis.**

With severe headaches associated with meningeal irritation (eg neck stiffness even in the absence of reduced consciousness and focal neurological signs) you need to consider meningitis and SAH and admit for an urgent lumbar puncture (LP) (once ↑ICP has been excluded by a CT scan).

SAH is caused by spontaneous bleeding into the subarachnoid space. The most common underlying cause of an SAH is berry aneurysms, ie aneurysms on the circle of Willis, eg middle cerebral artery aneurysm. An SAH causes ↑ICP resulting in reduced GCS; the blood also irritates the meninges, causing meningeal symptoms/signs.

Rob is rushed to the emergency department where on admittance his GCS is 7.

QUESTIONS
PAGES 58–61

List 6 causes of coma   *3 marks*

1. **Infection: meningitis, encephalitis.**

2. **Head injury (see Emergency medicine Case 1).**

3. **Vascular: SAH, CVA, extradural/subdural haematoma.**

4. **Epilepsy.**

5. **Drugs: CNS depressants including alcohol.**

6. **Endocrine: hypoglycaemia, ketoacidotic coma, hypothyroidism, hypoadrenalism (eg Addison's disease).**

7. **Metabolic: uraemia (renal failure), hepatic encephalopathy (liver failure).**

8. **Hypothermia.**

9. **Brain tumours.**

10. **Respiratory failure.**

🌀 Coma is defined as 'unrousable unresponsiveness' or a GCS ≤ 8 with no eye response. It is caused by either diffuse bilateral cortical dysfunction (eg metabolic) or damage to the ascending reticular activating system within the brain stem (eg brain-stem CVA, ↑ICP causing brain stem coning).

An emergency brain CT scan is performed which shows blood within the basal cisterns (subarachnoid reservoirs at the base of the brain containing large pools of CSF) of Rob's brain, confirming the diagnosis of an SAH.

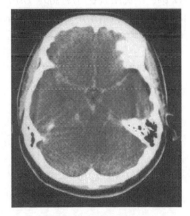

If Rob's CT scan was negative how would you exclude an SAH?   *2 marks*

1. **Lumbar puncture > 12 h after the onset of headache for xanthochroma.**

🟠 With small bleeds the CT scan may be negative. If it shows no mass lesion, intracerebral haematoma or hydrocephalus (all contraindications), perform an LP > 12 hours after the headache onset. With an SAH the CSF will be blood stained and yellow (xanthochromic as a result of the breakdown of blood). If CSF is blood stained but not xanthochromic, it is probably caused by a traumatic tap.

How do you prevent vasospasm after a bleed?   *1 mark*

Vasospasm follows a bleed causing ischaemia ± focal neurological deficits and is prevented by:

1. **Adequate hydration: fluid balance needs to be carefully monitored to prevent ↑ICP (causing secondary brain damage) and vasospasm.**

2. **Nimodipine (Ca²⁺ channel antagonist).**

🟠 Initial management of SAH involves ABCs, although blood pressure must be controlled to minimise the risks of a rebleed (a common cause of death). All patients should be referred for neurosurgical opinion about angiography (to detect site of bleed) and surgery (although surgery to clip the aneurysm is generally reserved for patients who are neurologically intact). Patients who are comatose or have severe neurological deficits have a very poor prognosis.

Rob is transferred to the intensive therapy unit (ITU) but as a result of the severity of his bleed continues to deteriorate. Several days later he is diagnosed as 'brain dead'.

Describe 4 of the tests used to diagnose brain-stem death   *4 marks*

Emergency Medicine

In brain-stem death (brain death) all brain-stem reflexes are absent:

1. Unreactive pupils, ie fixed and unresponsive to light.

2. Absent corneal reflexes: no blink response to stimulation of the cornea.

3. Oculocephalic reflexes are absent, ie no doll's eye movements: when head is moved side to side, eyes move with the head (with an intact brain stem the eyes move relative to the orbit).

4. No vestibulo-ocular reflexes: no eye movement occurs after injection of ice-cold water into each external meatus.

5. No motor response within the cranial nerve territory to painful stimuli.

6. No gag reflex in response to pharyngeal stimulation.

7. No respiratory effort: spontaneous respiration is absent in response to stopping the ventilator and allowing Pco_2 to rise to > 6.7 kPa.

🛈 Before diagnosing brain-stem death, it is necessary to establish that the patient is in an apnoeic coma and the absence of drug intoxication, hypothermia, hypoglycaemia, acidosis and electrolyte imbalance.

Rob is considered suitable for organ donation so his girlfriend and parents are approached for permission, because his wishes regarding organ donation are unknown.

List 4 patient criteria for organ donation   *2 marks*

For a patient to be considered suitable for organ (kidney, liver, cornea, heart pancreas or lungs) donation, the following criteria must be met:

1. Aged 0–75 years.

2. Has suffered brain-stem death.

3. Is maintained on a ventilator.

4. Has no known cancer.

5. Has no sepsis.

6. Has no risk factors for HIV infection.

❶ You may also wish to read the BMA paper entitled 'Organ donation in the 21st century: time for a consolidated approach', which is freely available at: www.bma.org.uk

Give 3 advantages of presumed consent   *3 marks*

The advantages of presumed consent, ie the patient is presumed to consent to organ donation unless he or she has registered objections, include:

1. **Majority of people would like to donate.**

2. **Would prompt more discussion on organ donation among families.**

3. **Rather than requiring the majority who would like to donate to carry a donor card or put their name on the organ donor register, presumed consent requires the minority who don't want to donate to register their objection.**

4. **It is more cost-effective to maintain a register of the minority who do not want to donate rather than the majority willing to be donors.**

5. **Relieves relatives of having to make decisions about donation during a difficult and emotional time.**

❶ You may also wish to read the BMA position paper on presumed consent entitled 'Human tissues and organs – presumed consent for organ donation', which is freely available at www.bma.org.uk

List 3 acceptable and 3 unacceptable criteria for receiving a transplant   *3 marks*

Acceptable:

1. **The likelihood of a successful transplant, eg donor and recipient tissue type (racial minorities are less likely to receive a transplant because they are less likely to have proper HLA matching).**

2. **The urgency of the recipient's condition.**

3. **The probable improvements to the recipient's quality of life.**

4. **The probable duration of benefit, eg the duration of benefit is likely to be greater in a child than in an elderly person.**

Unacceptable:

1. **Ability to pay.**

2. **Social worth, eg teacher versus a 'no win, no fee' solicitor.**

3. **Race: although this may be unavoidable with regard to tissue matching.**

4. **Perceived contribution to their own illness.**

5. **Past use of medical resources.**

Total: *20 marks*

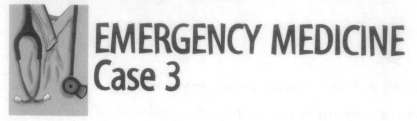

EMERGENCY MEDICINE
Case 3

Simon, a 69-year-old known patient with ischaemic heart disease (IHD), is brought into the emergency department with several hours' history of progressive shortness of breath.

What is the differential diagnosis?   *2 marks*

1. **Acute pulmonary oedema (acute left ventricular failure).**

2. **Exacerbation of airway disease, either asthma or chronic obstructive pulmonary disease (COPD).**

3. **Pneumonia.**

4. **Pulmonary embolus.**

5. **Pneumothorax.**

ⓘ Asthma/COPD, pulmonary oedema and pneumonia may be hard to distinguish and may coexist; if in doubt treat all three simultaneously, eg bronchodilators, antibiotics, diuretics (although pulmonary oedema/pneumonia should be confirmed on a CXR).

On examination he is clearly distressed, sweaty and pale with signs consistent with acute heart failure.

What are the signs of acute <u>left ventricular failure</u>?   *3 marks*

1. **Tachypnoea.**

2. **Tachycardia.**

3. **Triple or gallop rhythm: triple rhythm is the result of third or fourth heart sound. A gallop rhythm is a fast triple rhythm.**

4. **Lung crepitations.**

QUESTIONS
PAGES 62–65

5. **Cardiac wheeze.**

6. **Pink frothy sputum.**

7. **Cyanosis.**

8. **Cold extremities ('shut down').**

ⓘ Cardiac causes of acute pulmonary oedema include MI, ACS, arrhythmias and valvular heart disease. Non-cardiac causes include ARDS and fluid overload.

What is your immediate management?   *2 marks*

1. **High-flow O$_2$.**

2. **Furosemide (frusemide): 50–100 mg by slow intravenous injection.**

3. **Diamorphine: 2.5–5 mg by slow intravenous injection. This both sedates the patients and causes vasodilatation, reducing both pre- and afterload.**

4. **Antiemetic: to counteract the effects of diamorphine.**

5. **GTN (glyceryl trinitrate) spray: reduces preload (although use with caution in hypotension).**

ⓘ Also give 300 mg aspirin if you suspect that MI is the precipitating cause.

You request a CXR and ECG and take bloods for FBC, U&Es, troponin T and ABGs.

Parameter	Simon's results	Normal range
pH	7.24	7.35–7.45
PO_2 (kPa)	11.8 (on 100% O$_2$)	10–12
PCO_2 (kPa)	6.9	4.7–6
HCO$_3^-$ (mmol/L)	14.6	22–28
BE	-11.2	± 2

What do these ABG results indicate?   *1 mark*

1. **Mixed acidosis.**

ⓘ Normal pH is 7.35–7.45 so a pH of 7.32 is acidotic. It is mixed (ie metabolic and respiratory) acidosis because $P\text{CO}_2$ is increased, ie in keeping with pH change, and bicarbonate is depleted. Metabolic acidosis is caused by increased plasma H+ concentration as a result of hypoperfusion whereas $P\text{CO}_2$ increases as a result of impaired gas exchange (although initially the $P\text{CO}_2$ may fall as a result of hyperventilation). Such patients may require ventilatory support on an intensive care unit if they fail to respond to the initial treatment.

Simon's erect AP CXR is shown.

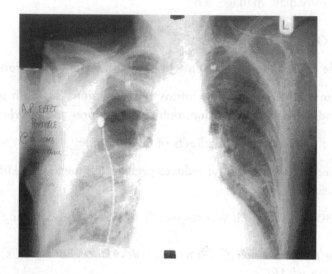

Identify 3 abnormalities on his CXR   ***3 marks***

1. **Alveolar oedema: diffuse shadowing extending out from both hila into the lung fields (Bat's wings), which is more marked on the right.**

2. **Fluid in the horizontal fissure: seen as horizontal line in the right lung field.**

3. **Upper lobe diversion: prominent pulmonary vessels in the upper lung fields.**

4. **Chest electrodes.**

ⓘ This is an AP film so can't comment on the heart size (AP films tend to make the heart look bigger than conventional posteroanterior [PA] films).

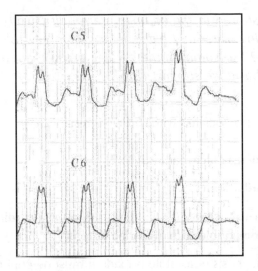

Simon's ECG (leads V5–6) is shown in the figure.

What does his ECG show?   *1 mark*

1. Left bundle-branch block (LBBB).

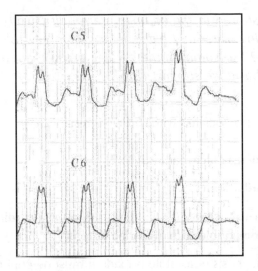 Widened QRS complexes (> 0.12 s), M pattern in V4–6 (the W pattern in V1 is often not developed), inverted T waves in lateral leads, ie I, aVL, V4–6. In the presence of LBBB can't comment on any other aspects of the ECG except whether the rhythm is regular or irregular.

How would you confirm that this is a new ECG change?   *1 mark*

1. Compare with a previous ECG.

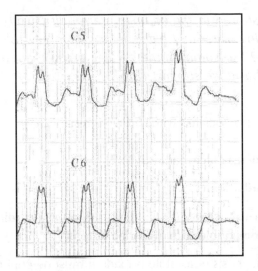 Simon is a known IHD patient so request his old notes in order to compare his new ECG against previous ECGs.

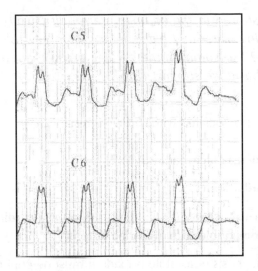 In the presence of typical chest pain, a <u>new</u> LBBB is an indication for thrombolysis (other indications for thrombolysis are ST elevation in 2 contiguous leads, ≥ 1 mm in the limb leads or ≥ 2 mm in the chest leads).

Emergency Medicine

187

Simon is transferred to the coronary care unit (CCU) for continuous ECG monitoring. Later that night he arrests in asystole. The nurse on duty dials 2222 to summon the cardiac arrest team and commences basic life support (BLS).

List 3 other rhythms associated with cardiac arrest **3 marks**

1. **Pulseless ventricular tachycardia (VT).**

2. **Ventricular fibrillation (VF).**

3. **Pulseless electrical activity (PEA): clinical signs of a cardiac arrest with an ECG rhythm compatible with a cardiac output.**

ℹ️ Whenever a diagnosis of asystole is made it must be confirmed by ensuring that the leads are attached correctly and checking the gain. Fine VF may be misdiagnosed as asystole; if in doubt treat as VF, ie defibrillate the patient.

How would you manage the arrest? **3 marks**

1. **Continue BLS: 15 compressions to 2 ventilations (although once intubated asynchronous, ie 100 compressions and 12 breaths/min).**

2. **Adrenaline: 1 mg iv every 3 min.**

3. **Atropine: single dose of 3 mg iv.**

ℹ️ Heart rhythms associated with cardiac arrest can be divided into two groups: VF/pulseless VT and asystole/PEA. The main difference in their management is the use of defibrillation in those patients with VF/VT. All patients should receive adrenaline 1 mg iv every 3 min. Also consider amiodarone 300 mg iv in shock refractory VF/VT (ie fails to respond after first cycle of three shocks) and atropine 3 mg iv in asystole and PEA associated with bradycardia.

List 8 potential reversible causes of cardiac arrest **4 marks**

1. <u>H</u>**ypoxia/hypercapnia: ensure adequate oxygenation/ventilation.**

2. <u>H</u>**ypovolaemia.**

3. Hypo-/hyperkalaemia and other metabolic disorders, eg acidaemia, hypocalcaemia: either revealed from recent U&Es or medical history, eg renal failure.

4. Hypothermia.

5. Tension pneumothorax: diagnose clinically (eg absent breath sounds on ventilation) and insert cannula into second intercostal space, midclavicular line to decompress, and a chest drain subsequently.

6. Toxic disorders, eg opiates.

7. Thromboembolic, ie massive PE.

8. Cardiac tamponade: difficult to diagnose clinically; suspect if penetrating chest wound.

🔴 During cardiac arrest potential causes or aggravating factors should be considered and treated as appropriate. For ease of memory these are divided into the four 'Hs' and four 'Ts'.

Give 4 situations where CPR (cardiopulmonary resuscitation) should not be attempted   *2 marks*

1. Where attempting CPR will not restart the patient's heart and breathing.

2. Where there is no benefit in restarting patient's heart and breathing, eg successful CPR offers only brief extension of life because co-morbidity means death is imminent.

3. Where the expected benefit is outweighed by the burdens: this is difficult to assess because it requires balancing the benefits of prolonging life against the burdens, eg side effects of traumatic CPR, prolonged hypoxia.

4. A valid advance directive refusing CPR.

🔴 You may also wish to read the following BMA paper available at www.bma.org.uk under the ethics section: 'Decisions relating to cardiopulmonary resuscitation'.

Total: *25 marks*

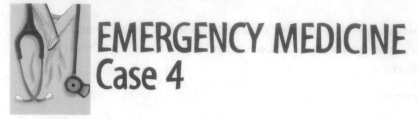

EMERGENCY MEDICINE
Case 4

Dan, an otherwise healthy 22-year-old student, is admitted to the emergency department with sudden onset of right-sided pleuritic chest pain and breathlessness.

What is the differential diagnosis?   **4 marks**

1. **Pneumothorax.**

2. **PE.**

3. **Viral pleurisy.**

4. **Pneumonia.**

5. **Musculoskeletal chest pain.**

① Pneumothorax is defined as air in the pleural space. It can be classified as primary, ie no underlying lung disease, or secondary (eg underlying COPD, asthma, lung cancer). The type of pneumothorax influences its management (see below).

Indicate (↑↔↓) the expected findings consistent with a pneumothorax   **3 marks**

Findings on the affected side

Breath sounds	↓ (decreased breath sounds)
Chest wall expansion	↓ (decreased chest wall expansion)
Percussion note	↑ (hyper-resonant percussion note)

① Pneumothoraces may be asymptomatic (especially if small) or present with sudden-onset dyspnoea and/or pleuritic chest pain. Patients with asthma/COPD may present with a sudden deterioration.

A CXR is ordered which shows a large right-sided pneumothorax.

QUESTIONS
PAGES 66–68

⊕ Pneumothoraces can be classified as small (<2 cm) or large (≥ 2 cm) according to the gap between the lung margin and the chest wall.

⊕ Radiologically a bulla may be misdiagnosed as a pneumothorax, although with pneumothoraces the visceral pleural surface is convex to the chest wall; with a bulla it is concave.

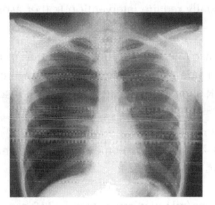

What radiological and clinical features would indicate a tension pneumothorax?

2 marks

Radiological:

1. **Shift of the mediastinal structures and heart away from the side of the pneumothorax.**

Clinical (signs of mediastinal shift):

1. **Tracheal deviation to the opposite side.**

2. **Shift of the apex beat.**

⊕ A tension pneumothorax is the result of air entering the pleural space on inspiration, which fails to escape on expiration, causing a shift of the mediastinal structures away from the pneumothorax. This will impair the cardiovascular system (CVS), causing tachycardia, hypotension and eventually cardiac arrest. It is a medical emergency made on the basis of a clinical diagnosis and is relieved by insertion of a cannula into the second intercostal space (ICS)-MCL (before requesting a CXR). A chest drain should be inserted immediately afterwards.

What action should be taken in Dan's case?   *1 mark*

1. Aspirate the pneumothorax.

ⓘ Management depends on whether the pneumothorax is primary or secondary. Small, asymptomatic, primary pneumothoraces can be simply observed; if symptomatic, aspiration is the first-line treatment. Secondary pneumothoraces usually require intervention (either aspiration or chest drain insertion).

ⓘ A pneumothorax is aspirated by inserting a cannula into the second ICS-MCL on the affected side. Stop if resistance is felt or the patient coughs excessively. The CXR should be repeated to confirm resolution of the pneumothorax.

Assuming his weight is 70 kg, what volume of 1% lidocaine can be safely administered (maximum dose 3 mg/kg)?   *2 marks*

1. 21 mL, ie 1% = 10 mg/mL; maximum dose is 210 mg (70 x 3).

ⓘ When aspirating a pneumothorax (or inserting a chest drain) you need to infiltrate down to the pleura with 1% lidocaine (not necessary if there is a tension pneumothorax). The first symptoms of lidocaine toxicity are perioral tingling; the patient may go on to develop seizures or cardiac arrest.

The CXR is repeated showing only a slight improvement in the pneumothorax with no improvement in Dan's symptoms.

What further action could be taken?   *2 marks*

1. Repeat the aspiration.

2. Insert a chest drain.

A 12-gauge Seldinger chest drain is inserted into the fifth ICS anterior to the midaxillary line and attached to an underwater seal. A repeat CXR 24 hours later shows expansion of the right lung field, although the pneumothorax is still present.

What action should be taken next? *1 mark*

1. Suction should be applied to the chest drain.

🛈 If the lung fails to fully re-expand (or persistent air leak), high-volume, low-pressure (-10 to -20 cmH$_2$O) suction can be applied to the chest drain. To confirm that the lung is fully re-expanded, a portable CXR (portable films to avoid detaching the constant suction pressure) should be requested, after which suction can be discontinued.

Should the drain be clamped before removal? *1 mark*

1. No.

🛈 You should never clamp chest drains inserted for pneumothoraces (especially if still bubbling) because, if the patient has a large leak into the pleural cavity, a tension pneumothorax may develop.

🛈 Chest drains may be removed 24 h after the lung has fully re-expanded and the air leak has stopped (ie tube stops bubbling), during either expiration or a Valsalva manoeuvre.

What advice should be given to Dan before discharge? *2 marks*

1. Pneumothorax may recur.

2. Avoid flying for 6 weeks: flying doesn't increase the risk of a pneumothorax but recurrence during a flight may have serious repercussions.

3. Diving should be permanently avoided.

4. Stop smoking: pneumothoraces are much more common in smokers.

This is Dan's second right-sided pneumothorax.

What further treatment should be advised? *2 marks*

1. Surgical chemical pleurodesis (with sterile talc) or pleural abrasion: this causes adhesions resulting in pleural synthesis, thus obliterating the pleural space.

2. Pleurectomy, eg via open thoracotomy.

Emergency Medicine

① Indications for surgical intervention: second ipsilateral pneumothorax, first contralateral pneumothorax, bilateral pneumothoraces, persistent air leak (> 5 days of tube drainage), spontaneous haemothorax, professions at risk (eg divers).

Total: *20 marks*

Further reading

British Thoracic Society. *Guidelines for the Management of Spontaneous Pneumothorax*: **www.brit-thoracic.org.uk**

NEUROLOGICAL CASES:
ANSWERS

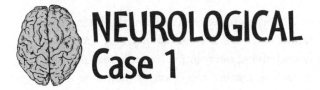

NEUROLOGICAL
Case 1

Mark, a 73-year-old widower, is referred to the emergency outpatient department by his GP with a 12-month history of progressive difficulty in walking and recurrent falls.

List 6 possible causes of falls in elderly people **6 marks**

1. Drugs, eg sedatives, alcohol.

2. Poor environment, eg poor lighting, loose rugs. Will require evaluation of home environment by occupational therapist.

3. Sensory impairment, eg visual impairment.

4. Musculoskeletal disorders, eg OA of hip.

5. Neurological, eg hemiparesis (CVA), Parkinson's disease, peripheral neuropathy (eg diabetes mellitus).

6. Syncope, eg epilepsy, vasovagal syncope (fainting), transient arrhythmias (eg third-degree heart block), hypoglycaemia.

7. Postural hypotension, eg secondary to antihypertensives or dopaminergic drugs, autonomic neuropathy, hypovolaemia.

8. Vertigo, eg benign positional vertigo (BPV), Menière's disease.

9. Drop attacks: sudden weakness of legs with no loss of consciousness (LOC), typically affecting older females.

10. Dementia.

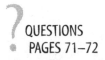
QUESTIONS
PAGES 71–72

197

🔘 The causes of falls in elderly people are extensive. From the history you need to elicit the exact circumstances of the fall, eg any LOC. You also need to enquire about any underlying neurological, cardiovascular and musculosketal problems as well as current medications including alcohol intake. Examination should include visual acuity, a full CVS examination with sitting and standing BP and the presence of any arrhythmias, and a full neurological examination.

As Mark enters the consultation room you note that he has a very slow, shuffling gait suggestive of Parkinson's disease.

What are the 3 main features of Parkinson's disease?   *3 marks*

The 3 main features of Parkinson's disease, which may occur in isolation or together, unilaterally or bilaterally, are:

1. **Tremor: see below for distinguishing features. May affect hands, tongue, lips and legs.**

2. **Rigidity: described as lead-pipe rigidity in limbs, trunk and neck. Cogwheel rigidity refers to juddering on extension of the flexed arm (caused by combined rigidity and tremor).**

3. **Bradykinesia, ie slowness of movement: causes slow shuffling gait especially when turning, expressionless face with reduced blinking, reduced fidgeting, quiet monotonous speech and micrographia (spidery writing). Bradykinesia can be assessed in the hands by asking the patient to simulate playing the piano and in the legs by tapping the heel.**

🔘 Parkinson's disease is a clinical diagnosis on the basis of its characteristic features (± resolution of symptoms on a L-dopa trial). Falls are also very common in Parkinson's disease and are often considered the fourth characteristic feature.

🔘 Typically patients complain of difficulty in rolling over in bed, difficulty in getting out of a chair, progressive slowing down (eg in walking, getting dressed) and deterioration in handwriting.

List 3 differentiating features of a parkinsonian tremor   **3 marks**

There are several characteristic features of a parkinsonian tremor that allow it to be differentiated from the other forms of tremor (ie intention and postural tremor):

1. **The tremor is slow (described as pill rolling of thumb over finger).**

2. **The tremor is worse at rest.**

3. **The tremor is reduced (or eliminated) on distraction.**

4. **The tremor is reduced (or eliminated) on movement.**

5. **The tremor is often asymmetrical (or even unilateral).**

🔸 Intention tremor: associated with cerebellar disease (eg multiple sclerosis [MS], CVA, alcohol misuse, anticonvulsants). The tremor is worse on movement, eg finger–nose test. It is associated with other features of cerebellar disease, eg dysdiadochokinesis, gait ataxia.

🔸 Physiological tremor: caused by exaggeration of the normal physiological tremor (eg anxiety, hyperthyroidism, drugs, eg β agonists, benign essential tremor, alcohol withdrawal). The tremor is fast, absent at rest and present on a range of movements.

🔸 Benign essential tremor is worse when the limb is in action, ie action tremor, and is partially relieved by alcohol. There is often a positive family history.

On the basis of the history and examination you confirm a diagnosis of Parkinson's disease.

Other than Parkinson's disease, list 2 other causes of parkinsonism   **2 marks**

Although Parkinson's disease is the most common cause of parkinsonism, other causes include:

1. **Drugs, eg neuroleptics (dopamine receptor antagonists), such as haloperidol (see Psychiatric Case 2) and MPTP (an impurity in synthetic opiates).**

2. **CVA.**

Neurological

3. **Severe head injury:** Mohammad Ali's parkinsonism is attributed to repeated head trauma.

4. **Viral encephalitis:** as portrayed in the film *Awakenings* (based on the book by Oliver Sacks).

5. **Progressive supranuclear palsy (Steele–Richardson syndrome).**

6. **Multisystem CNS atrophy (Shy–Drager syndrome).**

7. **Wilson's disease:** toxic accumulation of copper in the liver (causing cirrhosis) and brain.

8. **Westphal variant of Huntington's disease (genetic testing and counselling indicated).**

What is the underlying pathophysiology of Parkinson's disease?　　　*2 marks*

1. **Loss of dopaminergic neurons in the substantia nigra of the midbrain.**

🟡 The substantia nigra forms part of the basal ganglia (extrapyramidal system), which is responsible for the initiation and maintenance of fast, fluid movement. Parkinson's disease is a progressive neurodegenerative disorder caused by loss of dopaminergic neurons in the substantia nigra, which normally project to the corpus striatum using dopamine as the neurotransmitter (nigrostriatal tract). The corpus striatum still receives cholinergic (acetylcholine or ACh) stimulation that normally opposes the action of dopamine, but in its absence it causes inhibition of the motor cortex, resulting in parkinsonian symptoms/signs.

🟡 Dopamine itself is synthesised by dopa decarboxylase and inactivated by catechol-*O*-methyl transferase (COMT) and monoamine oxidase B (MAO-B).

Several months later mark is started on L-dopa, which greatly improves his parkinsonian symptoms.

What class of drug is combined with L-dopa to prevent peripheral side effects?　　　*1 mark*

1. Dopa decarboxylase inhibitor, ie benserazide or carbidopa.

🛈 The treatment of Parkinson's disease should be initiated by a specialist and not until symptoms significantly affect the activities of daily living. Typically first-line treatment is with a dopamine receptor agonist (eg bromocriptine, ropinirole) although eventually all patients will require L-dopa.

🛈 L-Dopa is a precursor of dopamine (which can't cross the blood–brain barrier) that is converted to dopamine by dopa decarboxylase, both peripherally and within the brain. It is given with an extracerebral dopa decarboxylase inhibitor to prevent peripheral dopamine conversion and its associated side effects, eg principally nausea and vomiting (caused by stimulation of the chemoreceptor trigger zone [CTZ]), which is treated with domperidone (extracerebral dopamine antagonist).

Name 3 complications of L-dopa therapy   *3 marks*

1. Postural hypotension on starting treatment.

2. Confusion, hallucinations.

3. Reduced efficacy (even with increasing doses).

4. L-Dopa-induced dyskinesias.

5. On–off effect: fluctuations in motor performance between normal function (on) and restricted mobility (off).

6. Shortening of duration of action of each dose, ie end-of-dose deterioration: dyskinesias often become prominent at the end of the duration of action.

🛈 Modified-release preparations and/or MAO-B inhibitors (eg selegiline) and/or COMT inhibitors (eg entacapone) may help the end-of-dose deterioration.

Total: *20 marks*

Neurological

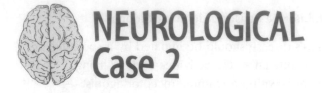

NEUROLOGICAL
Case 2

Jo, a 21-year-old student, is brought into the emergency department after having blacked out while watching TV at home with one of her flatmates.

Give 4 causes of <u>syncope</u>   *2 marks*

Syncope is the abrupt and transient loss of consciousness associated with absence of postural tone followed by a rapid and usually complete recovery.

1. **Vasovagal syncope (VS – simple faint): caused by bradycardia and peripheral vasodilatation in response to, for example, pain, emotion or prolonged standing.**

2. **Situational syncope, eg cough or micturition syncope: caused by reflex abnormalities in vascular tone and heart rate, which transiently reduce the blood supply to the brain.**

3. **Postural hypotension: LOC on standing from lying as a result of inadequate vasomotor reflexes. Defined as a drop in systolic BP of > 20 mmHg when standing compared with supine. Causes include drugs (eg antihypertensives, L-dopa) and autonomic neuropathy (eg diabetes mellitus).**

4. **Carotid sinus hypersensitivity, eg on turning head causes reflex bradycardia as a result of stimulation of hypersensitive carotid sinus baroreceptors.**

5. **Cardiac arrhythmias, eg AV block with bradycardia, sick sinus syndrome, VT.**

6. **Structural heart disease eg aortic stenosis, hypertrophic cardiomyopathy.**

7. **Transient ischaemic attack (TIA): caused by occlusion of vertebrobasilar arteries resulting in brain-stem ischaemia. TIA is a rare cause of syncope.**

8. **Hyperventilation, eg anxiety attacks. Resulting hypocapnia causes cerebral vasoconstriction.**

9. **Psychogenic eg hysterical, panic disorder.**

QUESTIONS
PAGES 73–75

What 6 questions would you ask Jo's flatmate <u>about the attack itself?</u>   *6 marks*

1. **Was there any loss of consciousness?**

2. **How long did the blackout last? For example, seconds in cardiac arrhythmia or minutes in epilepsy.**

3. **Did Jo lie still or where there any movements, eg jerky movements of arms and legs to suggest epilepsy? These are typically flaccid during VS.**

4. **Did Jo injure herself? For example, tongue biting is suggestive of epilepsy.**

5. **Any incontinence? Urinary incontinence is non-specific, faecal incontinence is suggestive of epilepsy.**

6. **Did Jo's colour change? Pale/green suggests VS, whereas pale then flushed on recovery suggests cardiac arrhythmias.**

7. **What was Jo's pulse like? Abnormal pulse in cardiac arrhythmias.**

Other questions you should ask include:

Before the attack:

(1) Was there any warning (aura)? An aura suggests epilepsy; nausea and light-headedness suggest VS; no warning suggests cardiac arrhythmia.

(2) What was she doing when it happened? For example, watching TV suggests epilepsy, prolonged standing VS.

After the attack:

(1) Any muscle pain? Suggests tonic–clonic seizure.

(2) How was patient after the episode? Rapid recovery with no confusion and amnesia suggests VS or arrhythmias; sleepiness with confusion and amnesia suggests epilepsy.

Jo's flatmate tells you that Jo suddenly stopped talking, fell to the floor and then started moving her arms and legs in jerky movements. Jo has no memory of the attack itself but says that she had no warning of it happening.

List 6 causes of seizures   *3 marks*

1. **Genetic: primary generalised seizure.**

2. **Pyrexia: in young children (febrile convulsion).**

3. **Alcohol: both intoxication and withdrawal.**

4. **Drugs, eg tricyclics; also withdrawal of certain drugs, eg benzodiazepines.**

5. **Metabolic abnormalities, eg hyponatraemia, liver failure, renal failure.**

6. **Space-occupying lesion, eg brain tumour.**

7. **Head injury.**

8. **Infection, ie meningitis, encephalitis.**

9. **CVA.**

🛈 Seizures are the result of abnormal electrical activity in part or all of the brain; convulsions are the <u>motor</u> signs of a seizure. Epilepsy is defined as a recurrent tendency to spontaneous seizures.

What type of seizure did Jo have?   *1 mark*

1. **Generalised tonic–clonic seizure (grand mal): as Jo experienced no warning (aura) the seizure was probably a <u>primary</u> generalised seizure.**

🛈 Epilepsy can be classified according to whether the seizure is caused by electrical activity occurring immediately within both hemispheres (primary generalised seizure) or within a focal part of the brain (partial seizure). Partial seizures may remain focal or spread to involve both hemispheres, causing secondary generalised seizures (see below).

🛈 Grand mal (tonic–clonic) is an example of a generalised seizure. The patient suddenly stiffens (tonic contraction) and falls to the ground with the limbs straight; there is no breathing during this phase, causing cyanosis (tonic phase lasts <1 min). This is followed by the clonic phase characterised by jerky limb movements (convulsions); there may be associated tongue biting and urinary and faecal incontinence (clonic phase lasts several minutes). The seizure is usually self-limiting, leaving the patient drowsy afterwards.

Give 4 features of temporal lobe epilepsy (TLE)   *2 marks*

The temporal lobe has a role in speech, smell and taste and memory. Focal seizures originating in the temporal lobe may cause:

1. **Sensation of déjà vu (undue familiarity) or jamais vu (feelings of unreality).**

2. **Memories rushing through the brain.**

3. **Hallucinations of smell or taste.**

4. **'Strange' sensations rising up the body.**

5. **Repetitive movement (eg lip smacking).**

🔵 The features associated with a partial seizure, eg TLE, depend on the location of the epileptic activity. In <u>secondary</u> generalised seizures these focal features may precede the generalised seizure and are termed the 'aura', ie warning to the patient of an impending seizure; in <u>primary</u> generalised seizures there is no warning (as in Jo's case). However, often the main indications that a seizure has a focal cause are the post-epileptic features, eg unilateral weakness (Todd's palsy) indicates a focal motor cause. When a patient presents with features suggestive of a focal cause for their seizure, underlying structural disease, eg SOL, must be excluded by CT or MRI.

What is the most useful investigation to confirm the diagnosis of epilepsy?   *1 mark*

1. Electroencephalogram (EEG).

🔵 During a seizure the EEG is abnormal showing focal (eg in the temporal lobe) or generalised 3 Hz spike-and-wave activity, confirming the type of epilepsy (partial or generalised). However, in about 60–70% of patients the EEG is normal between seizures (may also get false positives); the chance of detecting epileptic activity can be increased by repeat EEGs during sleep or by specific methods (eg hyperventilating or photic [light] stimulation).

Several weeks later Jo has a second seizure and the neurologist decides to start her on anticonvulsive treatment.

What is first-line treatment for Jo's type of seizure?   *2 marks*

Neurological

1. **Sodium valproate.**

🟦 Sodium valproate is the first-line treatment for <u>primary</u> tonic–clonic seizures. Carbamazepine is first line for partial seizures (± secondary generalisation). Newer antiepileptic drugs (eg lamotrigine) are recommended in patients who have not benefited from the older type of antiepileptic drugs or for whom they are unsuitable (eg poorly tolerated, drug interactions, contraindicated). Randomised trails comparing older and newer types of antiepileptic drugs have not found any difference in their effectiveness in seizure control.

What advice do you give women of childbearing age about antiepileptic drugs? **3 marks**

1. **Warn about interactions of antiepileptic drugs with the oral contraceptive pill (OCP).**

🟦 Some antiepileptic drugs induce hepatic enzymes and therefore increase metabolism of the OCP (both combined oral contraceptive [COC] and progesterone-only pill [POP]). A higher-dose OCP is recommended (50 µg oestrogen as a starting dose) or discuss alternative options (eg intrauterine contraceptive device [IUCD]).

2. **Explain about risk of untreated epilepsy during pregnancy.**

🟦 The main priority in pregnant women is to control her seizures because the risk of harm to both the mother and the fetus during a seizure is greater than the risk of taking antiepileptic drugs.

3. **Explain about the risk of teratogenicity with antiepileptic drugs.**

🟦 Antiepileptic drugs increase the risk of congential abnormalities including NTDs. To reduce the risk of NTDs woman should take 5 mg folic acid preconception and during pregnancy. They should also be offered α-fetoprotein (AFP) measurements and an USS at 18–20 weeks to screen for structural anomalies.

Total: **20 marks**

Further reading

NICE guidelines. *The Diagnosis and Management of the Epilepsies in Adults and Children in Primary and Secondary Care*: **www.nice.org.uk**

Neurological

PALLIATIVE CARE CASES:
ANSWERS

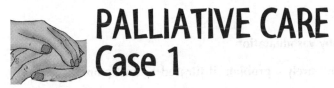

PALLIATIVE CARE
Case 1

Julia has breast cancer with bone metastases. She has had two recent hospital admissions for hypercalcaemia and is now on monthly pamidronate infusions. She takes diclofenac 75 mg twice daily (bd) and morphine sulphate tablets (MST) 120 mg bd for bone pain.

Describe the 3 steps of the analgesic ladder   **3 marks**

1. **Step 1: non-opioid (eg paracetamol, NSAID) ± adjuvant.**

2. **Step 2: weak opioid (eg codeine) + non-opioid ± adjuvant.**

3. **Step 3: strong opioid (eg morphine) + non-opioid ± adjuvant.**

ⓘ Analgesics should be given regularly because persistent pain requires preventive therapy. If the optimal dose of an analgesic fails to control the pain, move up the ladder, not sideways (ie don't simply swap to a different drug from the same class).

ⓘ Adjuvants include corticosteroids (used to reduce peritumoral oedema), anti-spasmodics (eg used to treat muscle spasm, bowel colic), bisphosphonates (used to treat bony metastases) and antiepileptics (used to treat neuropathic pain).

List 4 side effects of morphine   **4 marks**

1. **Nausea and vomiting: acts on the CTZ. Prescribe concomitant antiemetics, eg cyclizine.**

2. **Constipation: caused by decreased peristalsis. Prescribe concomitant laxatives, eg senna (stimulant laxative).**

3. **Drowsiness/sedation: tends to resolve after 5 days.**

QUESTIONS
PAGES 79–81

Palliative Care

4. **Dry mouth.**

5. **Hypotension: caused by vasodilatation.**

6. **Respiratory depression (rarely a problem if titrated against pain).**

7. **Addiction (again rarely a problem in palliative care).**

8. **Pruritus.**

Typical starting dose for morphine is 5–10 mg four times daily (qds) titrating upwards by 30–50% each time (accounting for previous weak opioid use). Once pain is controlled convert to a modified-release preparation, eg MST, which is prescribed twice daily (Σ daily morphine/2).

As pain is a physiological antagonist to the CNS depressant effects of opioids, morphine rarely causes respiratory depression.

Why should morphine be used with caution in renal failure?   *1 mark*

1. **May cause an overdose: reverse with naloxone (although this also reverses all of the patient's pain control).**

2. **May cause myoclonus.**

Morphine is metabolised to morphine-3-glucuronide (M3G) and -6-glucuronide (M6G). Both metabolites are excreted via the kidneys; morphine should be used with caution in renal failure because it may cause an overdose (as a result of accumulation of M6G) and myoclonus (as a result of accumulation of M3G). Fentanyl is the drug of choice in renal failure.

Unfortunately, her condition has deteriorated rapidly over the last week and she is admitted to St John's Hospice. She is nauseous with occasional vomiting, in obvious pain and unable to take oral medications.

Convert her oral morphine to 24-h diamorphine subcutaneous (sc) infusion   *2 marks*

1. **80 mg diamorphine, ie 240 mg/3=80 mg.**

🜊 Diamorphine is more soluble than morphine and is the preferred choice for parenteral administration, eg via a syringe driver. To convert oral morphine to parenteral diamorphine: Σ morphine/3.

🜊 Another possible form of analgesia in patients unable to take oral medicines is fentanyl patches.

Give 4 potential causes of Julia's nausea and vomiting   **4 marks**

1. **Drugs, eg morphine, chemotherapy.**

2. **Metabolic, eg hypercalcaemia, uraemia.**

3. **↑ICP as a result of brain metastases.**

4. **GI causes, eg gastric stasis (delayed gastric emptying) or intestinal obstruction (eg constipation, tumour).**

🜊 Vomiting is controlled by the vomiting centre (VC) in the brain stem which receives input from the cortex (eg ↑ICP), GI tract (eg obstruction), CTZ (eg drugs, metabolic) and vestibular apparatus (eg Menière's disease).

🜊 It is important to determine the cause of the nausea and vomiting because this will determine which antiemetic to prescribe (see below).

Julia is prescribed metoclopramide for her nausea and vomiting.

Where does metoclopramide exert its antiemetic effect?   *1 mark*

1. **GI tract: prokinetic antiemetic used to treat nausea and vomiting because of gastric stasis and functional bowel obstruction (contraindicated in mechanical obstruction).**

🜊 Other commonly used antiemetics include haloperidol (acts on CTZ), cyclizine (acts on VC), hyoscine (anticholinergic that acts as an anti-secretory/anti-spasmodic on the GI tract) and ondansetron (serotonin [5HT] receptor antagonist that acts on the GI tract and CNS).

Palliative Care

🔹 Some patients will require more than one antiemetic; however, anticholinergics block the cholinergic pathway through which prokinetic drugs act and so cyclizine (which has both antihistaminergic and anticholinergic actions) will antagonise the actions of metoclopramide on the GI tract.

It is clear that Julia is terminally ill and it is decided to no longer treat her hypercalcaemia.

List 4 factors that need to be considered when deciding to withdraw treatment   *2 marks*

1. **The current condition of the patient.**

2. **The risks (eg side effects) and benefits (eg improved quality of life, increased survival) of the treatment.**

3. **The views of the patient, eg a valid advance directive.**

4. **The views of the patient's family and relatives: although not legally binding they should be taken into account.**

5. **The views of the health professionals involved in the patient's care.**

🔹 Decisions to withhold or withdraw treatment on the basis that it is not providing a benefit to the patient should be made by the doctor with overall responsibility for the patient's care, taking into account the above.

🔹 You may also wish to read the BMA paper entitled 'Withholding and withdrawing life prolonging medical treatment', which is freely available at www.bma.org.uk under the ethics section.

Despite the analgesia Julia still continues to experience breakthrough pain. The nurse is reluctant to prescribe diamorphine as needed (prn) for fear of hastening Julia's death.

Give 3 reasons why such treatment is not considered to be euthanasia   *3 marks*

To distinguish between treatments primarily intended to harm patients and treatments that may harm patients when not the intended outcome, the following must apply (termed the doctrine of double effect):

1. The treatment is appropriate to the condition that it is intended to treat: diamorphine is appropriate analgesia for severe pain.

2. The treatment intends the desired outcome even if the harmful effect is foreseen: the aim of the diamorphine is to control Julia's pain even though it may hasten her death.

3. The harmful effect is not the means of achieving the desired outcome: the aim is to control Julia's pain through effective analgesia and not by killing her.

4. The benefits of the intended outcome outweigh any potential harmful effects: Julia is terminally ill so it is important to make her as comfortable as possible even if it unintentionally hastens her death.

Total: *20 marks*

Further reading

Each hospital should have its own 'care of the dying' pathway.

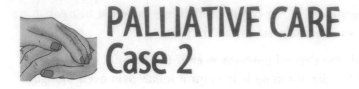

PALLIATIVE CARE
Case 2

Michael, a 72-year-old farmer, visits his GP complaining of several months' history of worsening back pain which is now no longer eased by paracetamol.

List 4 sinister back pain symptoms **4 marks**

1. **Non-mechanical back pain.**

2. **Localised bony tenderness.**

3. **Systemic features, eg weight loss.**

4. **Disturbance of bladder and/or bowel function.**

5. **Erectile dysfunction.**

6. **Saddle anaesthesia.**

7. **Weak legs/gait disturbance.**

ⓘ These symptoms may indicate a sinister underlying cause for the back pain requiring further investigation (see below). Symptoms (4–7) indicate cord compression/cauda equina syndrome requiring urgent referral (see below).

Name 4 primary cancers that metastasise to bone **2 marks**

1. **Lung.**

2. **Breast.**

3. **Prostate.**

4. **Thyroid.**

5. **Kidney.**

QUESTIONS
PAGES 82–85

① When investigating metastatic bone disease ALP (a marker of new bone formation) is raised, ESR is raised, calcium may be raised (as a result of metastases or tumour secretion of parathyroid hormone [PTH]-related protein), skeletal X-rays may show osteolytic (or osteosclerotic with prostate metastases) lesions and radiolabelled bone scans will detect bony metastases as areas of increased bone activity (often before radiological changes become evident).

The GP requests a number of outpatient investigations as below.

Investigation	Michael's result	Normal range	Investigation	Michael's result	Normal range
Hb (g/dL)	11.2	13–18	Na$^+$ (mmol/L)	142	135–145
MCV (fL)	91	76–96	K$^+$ (mmol/L)	4.1	3.5–5
WCC (x 10^9/L)	7	4–11	Urea (mmol/L)	6.6	2.5–6.7
Platelets (x 10^9/L)	220	150–400	Creatinine (µmol/L)	138	70–120
ESR (mm/h)	89	<30	Ca^{2+} (mmol/L)	2.7	2.12–2.65
			Proteins (g/L)	72	60–80
Urine dipstick	Protein	+++	Albumin (g/l)	25	35–50
Spinal X-ray	No vertebral fracture		ALP (IU/L)	70	30–150
PSA (µg/L)	3.4	<4			

ALP, alkaline phosphatase; ALT, alanine transaminase; ESR, erythrocyte sedimentation rate; Hb, haemoglobin; MCV, mean cell volume; PSA, prostate-specific antigen; WCC, white cell count.

Suspecting that myeloma is the cause of his back pain, Michael's GP refers him to the haematologists where the diagnosis is confirmed.

List 2 myeloma diagnostic criteria   *2 marks*

Myeloma is diagnosed on the basis of two of the following three criteria:

1. **Osteolytic lesions (see below).**

2. **Paraprotein in serum and/or urine: detected by electrophoresis.**

3. **> 10% plasma cells in the bone marrow.**

🛈 Myeloma is a malignant proliferation of plasma cells (antibody-secreting B cells) within the bone marrow that secrete monoclonal immunoglobulin (IgG or IgA) in the serum (paraprotein – hence, despite a low albumin, serum proteins remain within range). The abnormal plasma cells may also secrete free light chains which are secreted in the urine as Bence Jones proteins (hence dipstick positive for proteinuria).

🛈 Presenting features include bone pain and related features (see below), anaemia, renal failure (resulting from Bence Jones proteins) and infections (caused by impaired humoral immunity).

What does his lateral skull X-ray show?   *1 mark*

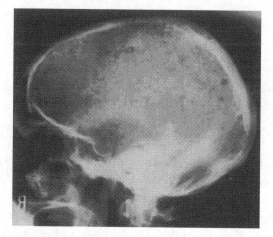

1. Multiple osteolytic lesions, ie pepperpot skull.

🛈 Proliferation of plasma cells within the bone marrow causes localised osteolytic lesions resulting in bone pain, hypercalcaemia, pathological fractures and cord compression.

🛈 The diagnosis of myeloma involves a skeletal X-ray survey of skull, spine, pelvis, ribs, femora and humeri for characteristic multiple osteolytic lesions (although bones may appear normal or diffusely osteoporotic). Myeloma is purely an osteolytic bone disease (bone resorption without bone formation), so radiolabelled bone scans, which rely on new bone formation for uptake, are insensitive for detection of myeloma bone disease (and hence ALP is normal).

Michael is treated with melphalan (for his myeloma) and a bisphosphonate (for his bone disease).

Calculate Michael's adjusted Ca^{2+} *1 mark*

3.0 mmol/L, ie 2.7 + 0.3 (ie [40–25] x 0.02)

🕛 About 40% of calcium is bound to albumin. Normally total calcium is measured, which reflects both bound and unbound calcium, although only the latter is physiologically relevant. Total calcium can be adjusted for changes in albumin concentration (affecting levels of unbound calcium) by adding 0.02 mmol/L to the Ca^{2+} concentration for every 1 g/L that albumin is <40 g/L.

Give 4 symptoms of hypercalcaemia   *4 marks*

1. **Abdominal pain.**

2. **Nausea and vomiting.**

3. **Anorexia**

4. **Constipation.**

5. **Polyuria.**

6. **Polydipsia.**

7. **Confusion.**

7. **Tiredness.**

8. **Depression.**

🕛 Hypercalcaemia is common in myeloma and all patients are given bisphosphonates irrespective of whether bone disease is evident (as protects against progression of myeloma bone disease).

🕛 First-line treatment of myeloma in older patients is melphalan. Treatment is continued with monitoring of paraprotein levels, which initially decline (with improved symptoms and blood counts) before reaching a plateau phase. Treatment is usually stopped at this point, although eventually the disease relapses (indicated by rising paraprotein levels).

Palliative Care

217

Michael's myeloma enters into remission, his melphalan is stopped and he is monitored as an outpatient. Eighteen months later his myeloma relapses and he is admitted with suspected cord compression confirmed by MRI.

List 4 other causes of cord <u>compression</u>   *4 marks*

1. **Trauma, eg RTA.**

2. **Malignancy: primary (eg neurofibroma), metastatic bone disease.**

3. **Disc prolapse, eg cervical spondylosis.**

4. **Epidural abscess.**

5. **Haematoma, eg complication of LP in a patient on warfarin.**

6. **Atlantoaxial subluxation, eg in rheumatoid arthritis.**

7. **Syringomyelia: fluid-filled cavity within the cord**

🌀 Treatment of cord compression caused by malignancy may include steroids, radiotherapy, chemotherapy and/or surgical decompression.

Name 4 <u>motor</u> signs that you would expect to find <u>below</u> the site of a cord lesion

                                                                          4 marks

1. **Muscle weakness.**

2. **Spasticity (although initially affected limbs will be flaccid).**

3. **Hyperreflexia ± clonus.**

4. **Extensor (upgoing) plantars.**

🌀 Cord lesions will cause upper motor neuron (UMN) signs; muscle wasting and fasciculation are associated with lower motor neuron (LMN) lesions. Although cord lesions may be complete (causing bilateral upper UMN paralysis, bilateral sensory loss and loss of bladder and bowel function), more commonly lesions are incomplete.

● As well as interfering with function of ascending and descending tracts, a cord lesion will also cause segmental signs at the level of the lesion, eg LMN lesion signs in the affected myotome and pain, paraesthesia or sensory loss in the affected dermatome.

Total: **20 marks**

Further reading

British Society of Haematology. *Guidelines on the Diagnosis and Management of Multiple Myeloma,* **available at: www.b-s-h.org.uk**

PAEDIATRIC CASES:
ANSWERS

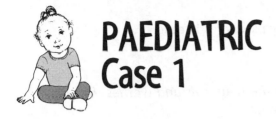

PAEDIATRIC
Case 1

Sam, a 2-year-old boy of African-Caribbean descent, is referred to Alder Hey after his mother has noticed that his fingers seem swollen and that he always seems tired. He is subsequently diagnosed with sickle-cell disease (SCD).

What is the inheritance of sickle-cell disease?   ***1 mark***

1. Autosomal recessive inheritance.

🖙 In SCD the patient is homozygous for the sickle-cell gene (*HbSS*). Both parents are heterozygous carriers (*HbSA*) and have a one in four chance of having a child with the disease (see below).

		Father HbSA	
		S	A
Mother HbSA	S	SS (SCD)	SA (carrier)
	A	SA (carrier)	AA (normal)

🖙 SCD is caused by a genetic mutation resulting in glutamine being replaced by valine in the β-globin chain.

What is the pathogenesis of sickle-cell anaemia?   ***2 marks***

1. In SCD the HbSS molecule becomes deformed (shaped like a sickle) in the deoxygenated state.

2. Sickle cells are more fragile with a reduced life span (10–20 days).

🖙 This leads to a chronic haemolytic anaemia episodically punctuated by crises:

- vaso-occlusive (infarctive) crises, caused by sickle cells becoming trapped in the microcirculation, obstructing blood flow to organs

- splenic sequestration crises, which can be fatal within hours

❓ QUESTIONS
PAGES 89–91

223

- aplastic crises, typically caused by parvovirus infection

- haemolytic crises.

Sam's mum is very upset about the diagnosis and worries that any future children will also be affected.

To where should mum be referred?   *1 mark*

1. Genetic counselling.

Genetic counselling involves giving parents information and advice (in a non-directive and non-biased manner) on inherited conditions. It aims to explain:

- the disease (e.g. clinical presentation, treatment, prognosis and complications)

- the genetics (e.g. the risk of developing symptoms and the risk to future offspring)

- reproductive options (e.g. antenatal diagnosis, terminations, in vitro fertilisation [IVF], adoption, ignoring the risk, not having more children).

Sam's mother is told that sickle-cell disease cannot be prevented but that it is possible to screen for it during pregnancy.

Give 2 advantages and 2 disadvantages of antenatal screening   *4 marks*

Advantages:

1. **Screening increases the reproductive choices of families at risk of affected pregnancies.**

2. **Some conditions identified through antenatal screening can be treated in utero.**

3. **A pregnant woman has the right to know if her pregnancy is at risk.**

4. **By terminating affected pregnancies it reduces future suffering.**

Disadvantages:

1. **Screening for particular abnormalities may encourage prejudice towards individuals with that condition.**

2. **Screening is not 100% sensitive and specific. It can create unnecessary worries if the test is falsely positive or false reassurance if the test is falsely negative.**

3. **Screening may reduce parental choice by expecting mothers with a positive test to terminate their pregnancies.**

4. **Screening may be used to identify pregnancies with conditions for which termination is unjustified.**

Now aged 4, Sam presents with a painful left hip and a temperature of 38.5°C. He refuses to weight bear on his left leg and mum denies a history of trauma.

Give 2 differential diagnoses   *2 marks*

1. **Vaso-occlusive crisis.**

2. **Osteomyelitis.**

3. **Septic arthritis.**

Vaso-occlusive crises may affect a variety of organs, including the lungs and bones. In infants, painful swelling of hands and feet (dactylitis or hand-foot syndrome) caused by infarction of the small bones may be the initial presentation of SCD. In older children and adults, painful eposides tend to occur in the long bones, hips, shoulders and vertebrae. The pain can last hours to several days or even weeks, and may be associated with a high fever.

Osteomyelitis, caused by *Salmonella* species in half of cases, may become established in infarcted bone and should always be considered in a child with marked signs of inflammation.

List 4 factors that may precipitate a crisis   *2 marks*

Paediatric

1. **Infection.**

2. **Dehydration.**

3. **Hypoxia, eg after strenuous exercise, high altitude.**

4. **Cold exposure.**

5. **Immobility.**

🛈 Management of vaso-occlusive crises involves analgesia (may require parental opiates), oxygen, fluids and warmth; any infection needs to be treated aggressively. Blood transfusions may be required during aplastic, sequestration and haemolytic crises.

Give 4 prophylactic measures important for SCD patients   *4 marks*

1. **Avoid factors that precipitate crises (see above).**

2. **Folic acid: increased demand as a result of increased RBC haemolysis.**

3. **Pneumococcal, *Haemophilus influenzae* B (Hib) and meningococcal C immunisations.**

4. **Prophylactic antibiotics, ie penicillin.**

5. **Hepatitis B immunisation: as a result of increased risk from blood transfusions.**

🛈 Infants and young children with SCD are at high risk of severe infection, in particular pneumococcal and *Haemophilus influzenae* sepsis, as a result of splenic dysfunction caused by repeated infarctions; as well as immunisations, they should receive prophylactic penicillin from diagnosis.

Now aged 9, Sam's condition has markedly deteriorated as a result of numerous, severe crises and it is now decided that he should have regular blood transfusions.

Give 4 acute complications of blood transfusions   *4 marks*

1. **Acute haemolytic reactions: incompatible transfused RBCs react with the patient's own anti-A or anti-B antibodies causing haemolysis, acute renal failure and disseminated intravascular coagulation (DIC). Symptoms, which present within minutes, include agitation, fever, hypotension, tachycardia,**

abdominal/chest pain and bleeding from puncture sites.

2. **Allergic reaction:** urticaria and pruritus within minutes of starting the transfusion are common (can simply slow down transfusion and give antihistamines), although rarely anaphylaxis may occur.

3. **Fluid overload:** a result of either too much fluid being transfused or the transfusion being too rapid. May cause acute left ventricular failure (LVF), eg tachypnoea, hypotension, tachycardia.

4. **Transfusion-related acute lung injury (TRALI):** transfusion is followed by rapid onset of breathlessness and non-productive cough.

5. **Infusion of blood contaminated by bacteria:** can cause a very severe acute reaction with rapid onset of hypotension, rigors and collapse.

⟐ As a result of similar presenting features, it is often impossible to identify immediately the cause of an acute transfusion reaction. In the event of a severe acute reaction, stop the transfusion, keep line open with 0.9% saline, re-check patient identity against name on unit, closely monitor patient (temperature, BP, HR, RR, SaO_2), and summon a haematologist.

⟐ Repeated blood transfusions suppress HbS production (vaso-occlusive crises are prevented if HbS < 30%), although this may result in iron overload (which can cause liver and heart damage) and alloimmunisation against donated RBCs.

Give 5 long-term complications of SCD   *5 marks*

1. Short stature and delayed puberty.

2. Chronic leg ulceration.

3. Gallbladder disease: caused by excessive bilirubin production secondary to chronic haemolysis.

4. Cardiomyopathy/heart failure: resulting from chronic anaemia.

5. Renal impairment: the kidney is prone to damage from sickle cells. Failure to concentrate urine predisposes to dehydration and crises.

6. Chronic lung disease, eg pulmonary fibrosis.

7. Cerebrovascular accident (CVA): caused by a vaso-occlusive crisis.

Paediatric

8. **Visual impairment: resulting from proliferative retinopathy.**

9. **Bone necrosis, eg avascular necrosis of the femoral head, osteomyelitis.**

10. **Psychological problems, eg pain in SCD can be so severe and debilitating that it interferes with school performance or employment and may also lead to opiate dependence.**

Total: *25 marks*

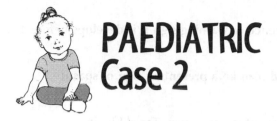

PAEDIATRIC
Case 2

Charlie is a 1-year-old, happy and thriving little girl. However, mum attends the community health centre because she is a bit worried that Charlie is a bit 'behind' all her friends. The health visitor carries out a development screening test noting the following:

Gross motor: **Good head control, sits with support but not by herself, hasn't started crawling yet**

Fine motor and vision: **Follows an object, reaches out to grasp, transfers toys with right hand to mouth, points with right index finger and has a good palmar grasp. During the test she doesn't use her left hand, which is kept closed**

Hearing and speech: **Turns to sound of name, vocalises when she is on her own, uses mummy and daddy and can say two to three more words**

Social behaviour and play: **She smiles, puts everything into her mouth, waves bye-bye and tries drinking from a cup**

What are the worrying features in this assessment? *3 marks*

She has delayed motor milestones, namely:

1. **Unable to sit unsupported (median age is 6–8 months).**

2. **Hasn't started crawling yet (median age is 8–9 months).**

? QUESTIONS
• PAGES 92–94

3. She has developed a hand preference (a warning sign if it develops before 1 year of age).

4. She shows fisting of her left hand (can be a presenting sign of spastic hemiplegia).

🟦 There is no delay in the other areas of development. The difficulty drinking from a cup is most likely a result of her reluctance to use her left hand.

As part of her assessment the health visitor also checks Charlie's immunisation status.

What immunisations should Charlie have had and when?   *3 marks*

1. **Diphtheria, tetanus, pertussis (DTP), Hib, meningitis C and polio vaccine. (½ mark each)**

2. **These are given at 2, 3 and 4 months of age. (1 mark)**

🟦 Her next immunisation is the MMR vaccine (measles, mumps and rubella). This is given at about 15 months of age.

The health visitor is worried that Charlie may have cerebral palsy.

Name 6 other clinical features of cerebral palsy (CP)   *6 marks*

1. **Dysmorphic features, eg microcephaly.**

2. **Failure to thrive.**

3. **Difficulty feeding: poor suck, poorly coordinated swallowing, vomiting.**

4. **Abnormal tone, eg hypertonic in spastic CP.**

5. **Abnormal posture, eg scissoring of the legs in spastic CP when picked up.**

6. **Abnormal movements, eg abnormal gait once walking is achieved, choreoathetosis.**

7. **Seizures: occur in about 30% of children with CP.**

8. **Persistence of primitive reflexes, e.g. Moro reflex: when there is sudden slight dropping of supported infant's head in the supine position, the hands open and arms extend and abduct, followed by arm flexion and cry. The Moro reflex is present at birth and should disappear by 6 months.**

9. **Hearing loss.**

10. **Visual impairment and squint.**

11. **Language and speech problems.**

12. **Learning impairment.**

🔵 Cerebral palsy signs evolve with brain maturation and growth and development. Cerebral palsy is the most common motor disorder in children, affecting 2–3 per 1000 children. About 50% of the children are diagnosed by 6 months and 70% by 1 year.

List 6 causes of cerebral palsy   *3 marks*

1. **Antenatal: cerebral malformation, fetal hypoxia, congenital infection (eg rubella, cytomegalovirus, toxoplasmosis), chromosomal/genetic disorders.**

2. **Perinatal: birth asphyxia (causing encephalopathy, although most babies who suffer birth asphyxia do not develop CP), birth trauma, hypoglycaemia, kernicterus, prematurity.**

3. **Postnatal: intraventricular haemorrhage, head trauma (eg non-accidental injury), meningitis/encephalitis, asphyxia (eg near drowning, choking).**

🔵 The most common causes of CP are antenatal causes (accounting for 80% of all cases), although often the underlying cause is unknown.

Over the next year Charlie starts to walk but Mum notices that her left leg is stiff, and when she walks she walks on tiptoes as she cannot put her left foot flat on the floor.

What clinical type of cerebral palsy has Charlie developed?   *2 marks*

1. **Spastic (1) hemiplegia (1).**

Paediatric

❶ Spastic CP is the most common type of CP (70% of cases). It may be in the form of hemiplegia, diplegia (mainly affects both legs) and quadriplegia (affects all four limbs and trunk). In spastic hemiplegia there is unilateral involvement of the arm and leg; often the arm is more affected than the leg. It usually presents at 6–12 months of age, often with early hand preference and reduced movements of the affected side. The child has a typical posture, ie arm is flexed and pronated and there is fisting of the hand; furthermore the child walks tiptoe (toe–heel gait) on the affected side.

❶ Other types of CP are:

- Ataxic cerebral palsy (10% of cases): caused by damage to the cerebellum; initially presents with (often symmetrical) reduced tone and delayed motor milestones, later developing poor coordination and balance.

- Dyskinetic cerebral palsy (10% of cases): caused by damage to the extrapyramidal pathways, leading to involuntary movements (eg chorea), poor postural control and dysarthria.

- Mixed pattern (10%).

What other features of this motor pattern may you find on examining her left leg?   *4 marks*

Spastic CP is caused by an UMN lesion, which is characterised by:

1. **Increased limb tone (spasticity): there is a resistance to passive movement, which sometimes can be suddenly overcome (clasp-knife effect).**

2. **Weakness (of dorsiflexors).**

3. **Brisk tendon reflexes.**

4. **Clonus: on rapid passive dorsiflexion of the ankle there is alternate involuntary muscle contraction causing repeated (more than five) plantar flexor movements.**

5. **Extensor plantar response: this is also called a positive Babinski sign. There is dorsiflexion of the big toe in response to a stimulus applied to the sole of the foot (eg scraping a pen along the sole of the foot). A normal response is plantar flexion of the big toe.**

🛈 There is no muscle wasting or fasciculation with a UMN lesion.

Charlie is referred to the child development service for assessment and management of her CP.

List 4 members of the child development team   **4 marks**

1. **Paediatrician.**

2. **Physiotherapist/orthopaedic surgeon: to optimise posture and mobility and prevent/correct skeletal deformities.**

3. **Occupational therapist.**

4. **Speech and language therapist.**

5. **Psychologist: to help manage associated behavioural problems.**

6. **Social worker.**

7. **Community nurse or specialist health visitor.**

🛈 The aim of the child development service is to identify the child's abilities and difficulties and subsequently formulate a plan to help the CP child develop to his or her full potential.

Total: **25 marks**

INDEX

*This index covers the answer section only. Page numbers in **bold** indicate the main subject(s) of each case.*

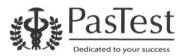